The Ten Best Tools

to Boost Your

Immune System

The Ten Best Tools

ELINOR LEVY, PH.D.

to Boost Your

and TOM MONTE

Immune System

HOUGHTON MIFFLIN COMPANY

Boston   New York   1997

For information about permission to reproduce selections
from this book, write to Permissions, Houghton Mifflin
Company, 215 Park Avenue South, New York,
New York 10003.

For information about this and other Houghton Mifflin trade
and reference books and multimedia products, visit The
Bookstore at Houghton Mifflin on the World Wide Web
at http://www.hmco.com/trade/.

Library of Congress Cataloging-in-Publication Data
Levy, Elinor
The ten best tools to boost your immune system / Elinor
Levy and Tom Monte.
p.   cm.
Includes bibliographical references.
ISBN 0-395-69460-4
1. Health. 2. Natural immunity. 3. Nutrition. 4. Health
behavior   I. Monte, Tom. II. Title.
RA776.5.L45   1996
613 — DC20   96-34239   CIP

Printed in the United States of America

Book design by Joyce C. Weston

QUM 10 9 8 7 6 5 4 3 2 1

Contents

PART III: SCIENTIFIC EVIDENCE

AND IMMUNE SYSTEM BOOSTERS

PART I

How Your Immune System Works

CHAPTER ONE

The Power to Heal Is Within You

WITHIN YOU LIES AN army composed of millions of soldiers, each one poised and ready to do battle for a single, overriding cause: to protect and sustain your life. It fights every single threat to your existence — bruises, burns, the common cold, cancer, cardiovascular disease, infections — even the harmful effects of your own behavior. And day after day, year after year, it wins. It is called the human immune system, and without it you wouldn't survive a month, much less sixty or seventy years.

Scientists have recently learned that the healthy functioning of this remarkable system is dependent upon your behavior. Certain behaviors clearly weaken immune response, whereas others make it stronger. In other words, whether your immune system is victorious against disease, or defeated by it, depends to a great extent on how you live. Researchers at the National Institutes of Health and major universities around the world are discovering that an array of foods, herbs, and lifestyle factors have a powerful effect on your immune system and consequently can improve your ability to fight disease. These nutrients and behaviors not only prevent disease, but in many cases also assist in the recovery from illness.

Unlike most common medicines, which deal exclusively with symptoms of illness, the new immune system boosters help prevent the onset of disease. They also play vital roles in helping your body stop cancer cells and tumors, even after they manifest themselves.

Scientists are also discovering that many of these boosters have a substantial effect. Researchers now believe that some of them can cut in half your chances of becoming ill. For those who are already sick, certain immune system boosters can promote recovery and may even extend life. Among the most important ones are the antioxidants, nutrients that stop the breakdown of cells and tissues that forms the basis for many diseases and for aging.

"For years, everyone thought the effect of these substances would be small," says William Pryor, Ph.D., director of the Biodynamics Institute at Louisiana State University in Baton Rouge. "I have been working on antioxidant research for twenty years, and even I used to say, 'Don't expect a lot.' But now we're finding there's about a 50 percent reduction in illness in many cases, and that 50 percent benefit is consistent. If we could cut chronic diseases in half by using nutritional therapy, we'd be making a profound difference, especially when you consider the cost of treating these diseases."

Nutrition and exercise are not the only potent immune system boosters available, however. Research is showing that meditation, relaxation techniques, and other ways to utilize the power of the mind to support the body also improve the ability to fight disease. Even the presence of intimate and supportive relationships plays a vital role in how well you fight disease.

This knowledge could be crucial to supporting and enhancing life in the modern world. Today we face new, powerful threats to our health. Some of the most dangerous ones include the human immunodeficiency virus (HIV), new strains of bacteria that are resistant to antibiotics, unprecedented levels of environmental pollution, and equally unprecedented quantities of dietary toxins. Any one of these can destroy life, but all of them together present a formidable threat to human health.

Many apparently new, mysterious diseases like *Ebola* virus for which science has no cure are now emerging. At the same time, several old diseases are becoming unresponsive to formerly reliable treatments and drugs, such as antibiotics. (Many of these antibiotics also depress the immune system, which means that long-term use may be counterproductive to long-term health.) Finally, some microorganisms such as the AIDS virus mutate rapidly, so that medicine cannot keep up with new strains of disease.

The best defense against old and new diseases is a strong, well-functioning immune system. Inside of you lies the most creative and formidable array of medical tools ever conceived — at least when it's healthy. The health of that system depends on you.

This book will give you new insights into the mysterious workings of your body and how your immune system defeats disease. It will show you how to keep your immune system fit and strong, which will help you boost your health and overcome illness. You will learn

- How much of a specific vitamin or mineral you should take
- Which herbs boost immunity and fight disease
- How much exercise and meditation you need to strengthen your defenses
- Which illnesses respond best to specific vitamins, minerals, herbs, and foods
- How you can use your mind to improve your health

The program offered in this book can boost your immune defenses substantially and can dramatically change the quality — and perhaps the quantity — of your life.

■ ■ ■

Some of the strengths and weaknesses of your immune defenses result from your genetic makeup, which you inherited from your parents and ancestors and cannot change. Yet scientists have discovered that lifestyle factors can also influence your degree of susceptibility and therefore may determine whether or not you actually contract a given illness, even though you may well be predisposed to it. Thus, even within our genetic limitations lies great latitude for building up our defenses. Unless your immune system is already thoroughly compromised or destroyed by an illness, it is within your power to strengthen or weaken it through your behavior.

Taking responsibility for our own health and adopting a lifestyle that actually boosts the immune system is a new way of thinking for most of us. Our society has been so used to turning to external means for healing — a pill, potion, or surgery — that it takes a certain reorientation to understand that we are responsible, to a large extent, for our own health. Most Americans believe that health derives from the knowledge of physicians — not from our own daily behavior. This strong belief is potentially disastrous. Our study has taught us that each of us creates the conditions that make the immune system strong or weaken it, allowing illness to take root.

Since the emergence of medical systems some four thousand to five thousand years ago, virtually all healing traditions have been based upon the idea that the body itself possesses "healing powers," and that, given the right assistance, it is capable of protecting itself against disease and healing itself of illness. The role of the physician is to promote the healing forces within the patient and thereby reestablish health.

Our modern medical system arose largely in the absence of such a philosophy. We based our approach on defeating illness by external means, through the use of pharmaceuticals or surgical intervention. In other words, we discounted the internal healing forces in favor of various agents designed to defeat disease.

Although it has provided great advances in scientific and technological understanding, Western medicine nonetheless has its limitations. A wide array of intractable illnesses, such as heart disease, cancer, and most recently AIDS, has forced us to reconsider our approach. Consequently, today we are more focused on the need to prevent disease before it manifests itself. The emphasis on prevention has also caused us to examine the means by which the body protects itself against disease and reestablishes health. The major system that performs that task, of course, is the immune system.

Since the advent of AIDS and the discovery of the human immunodeficiency virus, our knowledge of the human immune system has expanded by quantum leaps. We have developed the ability to examine the system on cellular and subcellular levels. We now know a great deal about how the immune system communicates with its trillions of member cells, and how these immune cells and proteins distinguish, say, a flu virus from your own cells, and then mount a perfectly balanced attack that destroys such antagonists before they can cause a single sniffle or passing nausea. And in a sense, our expanding knowledge and growing technical abilities have brought us full circle with the earliest pioneers of medical science. As we peer deeper into the world of cells and chemical messengers, we find ourselves confronting the body's healing powers — what we now call the human immune system. This book will acquaint you with that system and show you how to strengthen it in order to protect and restore your health.

CHAPTER TWO

The Miraculous Army

THE IMMUNE SYSTEM continually reveals itself as fascinatingly human, possessing many of the complexities and contradictions that characterize human behavior in general. For example, its tendency to kill cells that do not perform adequately might resemble some of the brutal behaviors of human beings. Conversely, its capacity to teach maturing cells to discern between substances that support health and those that are dangerous seems to reflect the human ability to instruct and to learn. The immune system continually generates incredibly creative solutions to an unpredictable array of challenges to human health. It can "think on its feet," endowed with an intelligence, power, and coordination that can only be admired.

In this chapter, we will see how much the immune system acts like us — not just "us" as individuals, but as a highly developed and integrated community. The immune system's community is populated by a collection of individual cells with specialized, yet well-coordinated tasks. Each of these roles is essential in protecting us from threats from our environment. Most remarkable is the system's coordination of its vast army of cells and chemical factors to effect a specific goal — to maintain that complex and delicate condition we call health. And it does this every day we are alive.

The Main Divisions of the Immune System

The immune system consists of a million million immune cells, a number that is beyond easy comprehension. Think of a million groups, each one composed of a million members. The system encompasses two different types of immunity: *innate* and *acquired.* Innate immunity comprises those abilities you were born with; acquired abilities are developed as you encounter various pathogens over the course of your lifetime. The immune system remembers every encounter with a bacterium or virus and is able to recall and reproduce an effective formula to destroy the invader, should it attack the body again.

Another distinction within the immune system can be made between agents of *cellular immunity* — those abilities that are rooted in cells — and *humoral immunity,* which refers to chemical factors that circulate in the blood and tissues. The primary job of the whole system is to protect you from infections from antagonists including bacteria, viruses, and various forms of fungi. It also plays an important role in protecting you from cancer. In order to do this, the system mounts an *immune response,* an incredibly complex process in which organized groups of cells and proteins combine to defeat a disease-causing agent.

A given immune response will depend upon the nature of the challenging agent, how and where it gets into the body, and whether or not the body has had a previous contact with that agent. Challenges within the respiratory tract will be handled quite differently from challenges through the skin. These responses, though often beyond your control, are influenced by behavior. For example, a response to an inhaled antigen in a smoker's lungs will be very different from the response in a non-smoker's, and this may account for the greater frequency of respiratory infections in smokers.

Like the nervous system, the immune system runs a highly effective sensory network. It has the daunting task of distinguishing what is *self* from *nonself.* It can differentiate between two proteins that each contain hundreds of amino acids and differ in only one of them. Anything the immune system recognizes as nonself is called an *antigen,* and the system is capable of recognizing many millions of different antigens. Recognition is the first step in initiating an immune response. Many different immune cells and components respond to a single antigen, but that individual response will represent only a tiny portion of the total pool of immune cells. In other words, the immune system usually gets the job done with only a fraction of its total strength.

The immune system can, however, backfire and attack essential human tissues. This response occurs in certain diseases such as multiple sclerosis, in which the immune system attacks the myelin sheath that covers and insulates the nerve fibers. But for the vast majority of people, the immune system accurately distinguishes self from nonself and reserves its powerful, destructive attack force for antigens that invade the body. How it is able to make this distinction will be explained shortly — at least to the extent that science understands it.

Military or police metaphors can help describe the behavior of the immune system. It employs cells that resemble highway patrols and others that approximate sophisticated law enforcement agencies, comparable to the FBI. Some of its units function like antiterrorist units, and still others collect information, as the CIA does. The system possesses both rudimentary and sophisticated weapons — in fact, some of them are more advanced in performance and reliability than those that current military establishments own. Its communication and early warning systems act like highly sensitive trip wires. Once triggered, these sensory systems both alert the overall immune system to the presence of an invader and attack that invader themselves.

Other metaphors are required to describe the full range of the immune system's functions. Its technical capabilities resemble the workings of advanced computers. Certain cells serve as teachers. Others exist as the system's living memory; indeed, these cells are sometimes referred to as "old wise cells." One of the organs associated with the immune system, the thymus gland, is actually a "school" in which cells are trained to recognize and deal with foreign invaders. Many of the system's abilities are not yet fully understood.

Let's begin our exploration of this community of cells and chemicals with the cells known as granulocytes, our first line of defense against an endless array of antagonists.

Granulocytes: The Highway Patrol Officers

Granulocytes are a type of white blood cell that forms part of a larger family of cells, called phagocytic cells. The least sophisticated of the phagocytic cells, granulocytes circulate in your bloodstream and enter your tissues at the first sign of infection. Like highway patrol officers, they protect certain areas from possible trouble that could spring up without warning. In this way, they maintain health in localized areas of the body. Like all highway patrols, they turn up at the accidents: the cuts, bruises, and places that are infected by bacteria.

Relatively unsophisticated in their ability to discern the types of "bad guys" they might encounter, granulocytes tend to be blunt and violent in their methods. In effect, they shoot first and ask questions later. Thus, when the skin is broken and the tissues exposed to dirt, bacteria, or some other foreign substance, the granulocytes rush to the scene and start ingesting everything in sight that looks suspicious. These ingested substances are destroyed by a variety of toxic chemicals produced inside the granulocyte's stomach, which is called a lysosome. The poisons it generates include hydrogen peroxide, nitric oxide, and hypochlorite (the active ingredient in bleach). Granulocytes literally digest the invader and render it harmless.

Granulocytes keep foreign invaders from gaining a foothold in the bloodstream, cells, and tissues. They cordon off an area of the body to keep the intruder and the resulting infection localized. Unfortunately, within that area they create havoc. Granulocytes often produce more digestive enzymes than are essential to destroy the antigens. Having produced these powerful chemicals in abundance, granulocytes sometimes release the toxic substances into the surrounding area, thus destroying healthy "innocent bystander" tissues. The result is the production of free radicals in the tissues and inflammation. When you look at a cut in your thumb, for example, and it appears swollen and red, you can rest assured that your granulocytes are shooting everything in sight — including the healthy tissues of your thumb. Don't be alarmed, however. The situation is temporary and relatively harmless.

Consistent with their "Dirty Harry" temperaments, granulocytes live short lives. They exist for a few hours or a few days and typically go out in a blaze of glory, diving into affected areas and being destroyed themselves in the battle against an intruder. Despite their sloppy unsophistication, granulocytes get the job done virtually every time they confront bacterial intruders that enter through the skin or lungs. What appear to us as tiny infections or minor irritations could potentially spread and cause a far graver illness. The granulocytes stop these infections in their tracks. And they do it with limited inconvenience to us.

Macrophages: FBI Agents and Servants of a Loftier Authority

A more sophisticated cousin of the granulocyte is the macrophage. Both granulocytes and macrophages are white blood cells, but macrophages can be thought of as the next level up in law enforcement — the FBI, perhaps. They possess the same weaponry that granulocytes do, but macrophages are also highly intelligent and capable of calling out more sophisticated reinforcements to deal with threats to the system.

Macrophages circulate in the blood but can also migrate into tissues whenever an infection or foreign substance infiltrates. They are also located at certain fixed sites, such as the kidneys, the liver, the lungs, and the skin. The macrophages at the fixed sites tend to have specialized abilities suited to the types of invaders likely to be encountered in those places. There are fewer circulating macrophages within us than granulocytes — about 100,000 versus ten million, respectively, in a milliliter of blood.

Macrophages identify bacteria by bumping up against them. Highly sensitive antenna-like proteins radiate from the macrophage's cell membrane. Once a macrophage touches a bacterium with this antenna-like projection, it can identify specific characteristics on the bacterium's cell wall. The macrophage can then send the information back to its memory banks within its nucleus, which in turn launches the macrophage into appropriate action.

When activated, macrophages produce an array of chemicals that act as powerful weapons against bacteria, viruses, and cancer cells. Among those chemicals are hydrogen peroxide, nitric oxide, and hypochlorite (bleach). These highly toxic chemicals actually oxidize microorganisms to death. (Forms of oxidation are all around us. Examples include rust, the browning of an apple, and the wrinkling of skin.) Once the chemicals come in contact with a virus, a bacterium, or a cancer cell, they begin to break it down. These oxidative chemicals cause the invading organism rapidly to decay, or age and die.

Scientists still haven't figured out how macrophage cells recognize viruses or cancer cells. As we will see later on, cancer often goes undetected by the immune system. This allows the tumor to thrive until it is fully developed and in a position to be life threatening. Viruses can hide as well, thus shielding them from the onslaught of the immune system. When cancer cells and viruses are discovered, the immune system is usually capable of destroying them, no matter how virulent either might be. As science learns more about how detection takes place in both cases, new forms of therapy can be created to promote recognition and thus destroy these disease-causing agents long before they have a chance to cause trouble.

When the macrophage recognizes bacteria, viruses, or cancer cells, it releases a number of chemicals collectively called cytokines, which can effect bodywide changes, such as causing fever and inducing sleep. Among those cytokines is tumor necrosis factor, which can destroy cancer cells and tumors.

Macrophages have a much broader responsibility for protection than do granulocytes. Like the FBI, macrophages communicate across the entire system; the granulocytes (like the local police) focus on specific locations. More important, the macrophage shares its information with T lymphocytes to generate a still more sophisticated and powerful immune response. The term *T lymphocyte* describes two specific kinds of immune cells, the CD4 and the CD8, and both possess the capacity to call forth other immune factors against disease.

Complement: The Private Eye

Unlike granulocytes and macrophages, complement is not a cell, but a family of proteins that circulate in the blood. It is the most important of the innate humoral factors of the immune system. Proteins — whether they come from plants or animals — are themselves composed of building blocks called amino acids. Amino acids serve as the physical body of complement. They also act as catalysts, or triggers, of chemical reactions when they encounter a harmful substance that invades your body.

Once complement recognizes a threat to your health, it binds itself to the invading organism and pokes holes in its cell membrane, thus causing its death. Complement also produces a byproduct that causes healthy blood vessels to leak. This resourceful ploy sounds an alarm within your body. In effect, complement alerts the rest of your immune system that something is wrong. Your body responds to that message by sending granulocytes and macrophages to the area, which, upon arrival, recognize the foreign invader. In this way, complement acts like a cagey private investigator who stumbles upon a nest of bad guys; realizing he is outnumbered, he sets off alarms within the building, alerting whole platoons of local police. This reaction explains the redness surrounding or infusing an infection.

Lymphocytes: Army Generals and Wise Teachers

When a macrophage recognizes an invader that it cannot handle alone, or when it sees that the combined strength of the initial defense is inadequate, it calls out reinforcements in the form of a type of lymphocyte, or helper T cell, called the CD4 cell. CD4 cells are often referred to as the generals of the immune system. They organize and integrate the many components of the system to respond to a given antigen. CD4 cells have the ability to produce some, and call forth other, powerful immune elements that can deal more effectively with bacteria, viruses, and cancer cells.

Before a CD4 cell can do anything, however, it must recognize the presence of a specific bacterium, virus, or cancer cell. In other words, it must be alerted to the fact that an antigen is present in the system. Once that happens, it can make an appropriate response that will include calling forth additional help. Thus, the moment when the macrophage communicates to the CD4 cell that a specific threat is at hand is one of the most important steps in the entire immune response — especially if the threatening agent can cause a serious illness. If the CD4 cell failed to recognize the presence of an antigen, the macrophage and other phagocytic cells would be left to deal with the invader by themselves. Thus the heavy artillery — most of the killer cells, B cells, antibodies, and advanced communications networks — would remain dormant in the face of an antigen. Also, key immune cells would not multiply; hence, the immune system would ultimately run out of reinforcements. Only the CD4 cell has the power to call into action these and other powerful elements of your body's defenses.

Remarkably, the cells themselves seem to realize the gravity of their roles. The macrophage cell attacks an invading substance, consumes it, and regurgitates a tiny part of the invader's protein. That piece of protein, which may be no bigger than a chain of ten amino acids, is placed on a cuplike structure on the outer membrane of the macrophage. That cup is a molecule called a major histocompatibility complex (MHC for short).

The protein-antigen now rests inside the MHC molecule. At this point, the macrophage offers up the antigen to the CD4 cell, as if it were handing an important message to a superior. In fact, hundreds of millions of macrophage cells are doing this at the same time — offering up tiny pieces of protein digested and prepared for the CD4 cell — in the hope that one CD4 cell will recognize the antigen and then call out a full-scale immune response. Now it is up to the CD4 cell to react. This is the moment at which the immune system will either rally or flounder.

The CD4 cell's reaction to the antigen is not automatic. In order for it to recognize the antigen being offered, it must have on its own cell membrane a specific kind of receptor capable of reacting to that antigen. In other words, the antigen and the receptor must fit like a lock and key. Any single CD4 cell is capable of recognizing only a single characteristic on an antigen, which is enough to identify that particular virus or bacterium and thus send the immune system into appropriate action.

As millions of macrophage cells continue to offer fragments of antigen-protein to the CD4 cells throughout the body, only a tiny fraction of CD4 cells respond. The vast majority do not have the appropriate receptor for that antigen. The receptors on each CD4 cell are created from genes that are shared by all CD4 cells. Each cell makes its own unique receptor from the available gene pool. Many million variations exist. Individual CD4 cells are actually trained to recognize self and nonself (or antigens) in the thymus gland, located just in front of the heart. There the CD4 cells create a specific receptor, and thus take on a specific responsibility in your immune defenses. Once a CD4 cell is trained and has its own receptor, it is sent into the bloodstream, alert to the presence of specific bad guys. Each CD4 cell will replicate, or divide, and form new cells. These offspring will have the exact same receptor as their ancestor, ensuring that whole families of CD4 cells with the same receptor are available to recognize a specific type of antigen anywhere in the body. Whether a flu virus turns up in your liver or in your blood, family members of CD4 cells with just the right receptor will have been scattered throughout your body to recognize the virus at any site.

Also, most disease-causing agents can give rise to more than one antigen, which increases the likelihood of the agent's being recognized. In other words, your immune system's chances of recognizing any antigen are pretty good.

Once the antigen is recognized by a particular CD4 cell, the general goes to work. Now the immune system blazes with activity, as if it were suddenly plugged into a highly charged power source. A call to arms is sounded, a web of communication lights up across the entire system, and a million million immune cells take up their posts and immediately go to work.

You, of course, are not aware of this. Instead, you suffer a particular illness — say the flu — with all its well-known, rather humbling discomforts. At the same time, cells turn on genes to produce unique chemical antidotes to illness. Among these are natural killer cells (another lymphocyte-like white blood cell), which can also attack and kill cancer cells, and attack the flu virus. Like macrophages, natural killer cells act instinctively. At the same time, cells communicate with one another to mount a well-orchestrated attack on the invader. Cells travel across distances that, considering their size, are vast. Phagocytic cells and complement attack pathogens in the trenches. Reinforcements are produced at staggering rates and inconceivable numbers. And all the while the system learns from its experience — and records the responses that work — so that the next time you encounter this virus, your system will have a ready plan of action. In other words, the action is better than anything Steven Spielberg or George Lucas could conceive of.

Recognition of an antigen is one of the most delicate and essential aspects of the immune response. If it does not occur, or if CD4 cells are weakened or destroyed — as in the case of HIV infection — the immune system's arsenal will be greatly limited and, in the face of a life-threatening disease, eventually defeated.

Once the CD4 cell recognizes the antigen, however, that cell immediately begins to replicate itself so that more identical CD4 cells — with this particular receptor — can be posted throughout the system. Cells that recognize the problem in your body and can best manage the immune system's response are soon being transported throughout the bloodstream to command posts from head to toe.

Cytokines and Interleukins: The Army's Messengers

Once it arrives at its post, the CD4 cell immediately does what any good general would do: it gives orders. It does this by producing a group of powerful chemicals, collectively known as cytokines, that in turn trigger an array of immune and metabolic changes in your body. Among these cytokines is a family of interleukins — interleukin-1 to interleukin-17 (or IL-1 to IL-17). Interleukins work independently and collectively to produce multiple effects. IL-1 causes immune cells to mature rapidly and thus become competent to fight pathogens or cancer cells. IL-1 and IL-2 produce inflammation, which among other things increases heat and blood flow to the affected area of the body. You experience this activity as aching pains in the joints and other tissues. In other words, it's part of the unpleasant side effects of a cold or another immune reaction.

IL-1 and interferon signal your brain to make you sleepy. Once you're lying flat on your back, your immune system can direct your body's energy to fight the invader. Other cytokines signal your body to produce fever as well, which may be a strategic action designed to make your internal environment less hospitable to infection. Still other chemical messengers regulate hormone production and control mood; the well-known grumpiness, irritability, and fatigue so familiar to those who suffer from a cold are the result of a well-coordinated attempt to get you to stop working, get plenty of rest, and avoid social interaction. No one wants to see you, and you don't want to see anybody either. Thus the immune system prompts you to take care of yourself and to isolate yourself from others.

Three cytokines — IL-1, interferon, and tumor necrosis factor — combine to perform other tasks. They change your metabolism to increase blood levels of certain immune-related proteins while decreasing levels of certain minerals, such as zinc. It isn't yet known why the body decreases zinc levels. It is known that zinc is essential to mounting a strong immune response. Perhaps these minerals would be entirely lost if the blood contained disproportionately high levels of them, because they would be filtered out by the kidneys and eliminated through the urine. To avoid this, the immune system may instruct the body to withhold minerals in the tissues, thus making them available to strengthen immune response against infection, virus, or tumors.

As blood flow increases, whole armies of macrophages, granulocytes, and complement arrive on the scene to destroy invaders.
Complement will directly assist in the battle against microorganisms, but it will also create leaky blood vessels and that characteristic redness that usually surrounds swollen tissues. This will
attract even more macrophages and granulocytes.

IL-2 also stimulates T cells to divide, producing more of these
fighters. If needed, IL-2 will also trigger production of tumor necrosis factor to fight cancer cells and tumors. It also stimulates
the production of gamma-interferon, which prevents viruses
from multiplying by interfering with their replicative machinery.
Still other cytokines cause macrophages, natural killer cells, and a
group of lymphocytes called CD8 killer cells to become more
reactive and aggressive in the face of an antigen.

Interleukins (IL-2, IL-4, and IL-6) and interferon stimulate, or
"turn on," cytotoxic cells, which kill virus-producing cells and
cancer cells. These cells include a subset of CD8 positive T lymphocytes, macrophages, and natural killer cells. Cytotoxic CD8
cells can also be directed against foreign cells or organs and
cause rejection of transplants. These three types of killer cells
work together, each using its special talents to destroy invaders.
Tumor necrosis factor can also directly destroy cancer cells.

Although these reactions have been observed and recorded,
much about the immune system still mystifies us. For example, some interleukins and interferon cause the body to increase
muscle breakdown. Scientists do not know why this occurs, or
what good it does in the course of fighting disease. We do know
that it happens as a result of immune system activity and results
in increased levels of nitrogen in the bloodstream. Beyond that,
we do not understand.

Like waving red meat in front of a pack of lions, interferon
incites natural killer cells to attack a specific target, or antigen.
And like lions, natural killer cells have a rather narrow range of
responses to a target: they strike with ferocious hunger and kill it.

They do this by attaching themselves to cell membranes that are producing virus and either bite down on the membrane or produce chemicals that destroy the cell. They can also attack cancer cells in the same way.

B Cells and Antibodies: Soldiers with Chemical Weapons

CD4 cells produce IL-4, IL-5, and IL-6, which stimulate B cells to confront the invader and produce antibodies — specific chemical antidotes to the disease. B cells come up with clever schemes with the panache of sting operations. It seems they like to embarrass the invader, too. Once they arrive on the site, they identify the antagonist and begin formulating chemical agents and strategies to destroy the pathogen. B cells create these chemicals by shuffling genes within their nuclei to produce antibody receptors that will recognize the antigen. When this receptor interacts with antigens and cytokines produced by helper T cells, the B cell starts mass-producing its antibody. (Antibody is also called immunoglobulin, a generic name for several classes of antibodies — IgA, IgD, IgE, IgG, and IgM — that can destroy a pathogen in a number of ways.)

One of the B cells' favorite ploys is to coat the invading organism with a kind of antibody that attracts macrophages and granulocytes (a process called opsonization). This is like putting honey on a villain and placing him in the midst of a den of bears. B cells can create an antibody that attracts complement, as well. Once the complement arrives, it pokes holes in the pathogen's outer wall. The pathogen leaks to death.

Another favored strategy of B cells is to cover a pathogen in a type of antibody that acts like glue. Whole gangs of pathogens get stuck together, which makes them more visible to the immune system and simplifies recognition. Hordes of white blood cells rush to the scene, and the resulting attack by the immune system is decisive.

Still another strategy is to coat a bacterium or virus with an antibody that prevents the pathogen from attaching itself to other cells. Unable to gain a foothold in the body, the pathogen is easily eliminated through the digestive tract or from one of the blood-cleansing organs.

B cells will subtly modify their genes until the most effective chemical antidote to an antigen is found. That antibody then will be produced in sufficient quantities to destroy the invader, after which its makeup will be recorded in the system's memory so that the next time the system confronts this particular antagonist, it will have just the right chemical antidote in its files. B cells and their antibodies often turn up in lymph nodes and vessels, where they work with complement and white blood cells to fight viruses and bacteria.

■ ■ ■

CD4 cells also produce cytokines that stimulate specific immune cells to multiply. Interestingly, only those cells that are directly relevant to the task at hand are increased in numbers. These include CD4 cells with the right receptor for the presenting antigen (as we saw earlier) and certain B cells that produce antibodies designed to neutralize the current invader.

Only the CD4 cells that recognize an antigen are immediately ordered by their own genes to produce a new receptor — like a baseball glove — on the exterior of their membranes to catch IL-2, the cytokine that will order these selected CD4 cells to reproduce themselves. Thus IL-2 stimulates only certain CD4 cells to reproduce, and not others. Only those CD4 cells with the "baseball glove" for IL-2 will catch the cytokine and be ordered to reproduce.

All subsequent encounters with that particular pathogen, say a chicken pox virus, will receive a much more rapid and effective response. Thus, even though you may be reexposed to a given threat, you won't get sick. This concept is the basis for immunization programs: vaccines ready you for a quick response to dangerous invaders so you will avoid the illness they would otherwise cause.

■ ■ ■

While these individual responses are occurring, a complex interplay takes place among the immune cells and cytokines to regulate immune activities. Some cytokines stimulate activities; others limit them; still others turn off cytokines when the illness has been defeated and the job is done. In short, your immune response will be strong enough to complete the individual task, but not stronger than necessary.

Though the immune system is composed of one million million cells — seemingly a more than adequate number — it does in fact commandeer other cells into its service. The CD4 cell can turn cells outside the immune system — such as those in your liver, lungs, kidneys, and bones — into soldiers, too. It does this by producing cytokines that transform somatic cells into scouts that alert white blood cells that they are needed nearby. These recruited somatic cells can also assist in presenting antigen; they can place digested antigen proteins on their cell membranes and thus signal macrophage or CD4 cells that an invader is at hand.

Viruses, Bacteria, and Cancer Cells: The Enemy

A virus (such as measles, smallpox, the flu, or the common cold) is an insidious and stealthy invader. It is not a living cell, but a parasitic organism that takes up residence inside the body's cells. A virus does not have enough genes (in the form of DNA or RNA) to reproduce itself. Instead, it commandeers your cells' DNA and orders your DNA to produce more virus and virus-carrying cells. Thus it hijacks the body's genes and uses them for its own purposes.

Many viruses change the membranes of the cells they abduct, which alerts the immune system to their presence. Once recognized, the virus and its abducted cells are an easy target for the immune system's arsenal. Natural killer cells and cytotoxic T cells can destroy the virus-carrying cells within your body and thereby neutralize and eliminate the virus itself. These T cells (cytotoxic CD8 cells) develop memory of the attack, preparing them for future encounters with this particular virus. Also, cytokines can attract macrophages to the virus-carrying cells and thereby enlist the macrophages in the fight.

However, the presence of all viruses is not obvious to the immune system. Some, like the herpes virus, can hide in the nervous system and lie dormant for long periods of time, sufficiently inactive to remain unnoticed by the immune system. The virus is present but latent, and it can sit in its hideout for long periods. If the immune system has been weakened, the virus can migrate to another area of the body, replicate, and cause symptoms. The immune system will then attack and destroy those actively infected cells, but some of the virus can skulk back to its shelter and remain undetected.

HIV has the same capabilities. It hides out in the brain, where the immune system is reluctant to attack for fear of damaging brain cells. HIV also takes up residence within the immune system itself. It hides in the macrophage and CD4 cells, and it eventually destroys the CD4 lymphocytes. Thus HIV in effect cuts off the head of the immune system, destroying its ability to coordinate an intelligent response to the virus.

Viruses, like terrorists, travel light (they are not even complete cells themselves), have the ability to move in small groups, and act with stealth and deception. Bacteria, on the other hand, are much more obvious to the immune system and therefore pose a less significant risk, for the most part. Bacterial infection can, however, raise havoc (such as when *Escherichia coli,* for example, gets out of the intestinal tract and into the bloodstream); some forms can even be lethal. But bacteria are less deceptive than viruses and consequently easier to deal with. Viruses are comparable to highly sophisticated terrorists, but bacteria resemble common criminals — both can cause problems, but one is a great deal more difficult to deal with than the other. Medicine has come up with a whole range of pharmaceuticals that effectively neutralize bacteria, but science has come up with nothing comparable to, say, penicillin to deal with virus. Yet no wonder drug can replace the brilliant performance of an effective immune system.

Cancer is also an insidious enemy. Cancers start when the DNA in a single cell mutates to allow the cell to divide unchecked. In normal cells, the process of cell division is very carefully controlled at multiple checkpoints. It usually takes several different mutations to make a cell malignant. But although consequences can be catastrophic, the mutations that cause cancer usually are the result of subtle changes in only a few of the cell's thousands of proteins. Most tumors grow very slowly at first. This makes the job of noticing the new cells among the many trillion normal cells a formidable task. It would be somewhat analogous to tracking down the Unabomber before he sent out any bombs. Yet the immune system is thought by some scientists to do this routinely. Macrophages and natural killer cells have an uncanny ability to detect and destroy cancer cells.

If unnoticed, the cancer grows larger and continues to mutate. Often small pieces break off the original tumor and migrate to different locations to start new tumors. This process is called metastasis. Often, by the time the immune system figures out the tumor cells are not law-abiding members of the community, the tumor has grown and spread. At this point the battle is on, but the outcome is uncertain. It depends on the strength of the immune system and the size and location of the tumor.

Shutting Down the System — Before It Hurts *You*

Once the immune response has defeated an illness, it shuts itself off. This regulation is largely accomplished by a particular type of T lymphocyte called a CD8 suppressor cell, which produces chemicals that slow down and ultimately shut off the immune response, usually by shutting down CD4 cell activity.

At times, however, the immune response can be too strong and can cause damage to healthy and even essential tissues. This is especially a concern with infections in the brain, where inflammation can threaten life; for instance, cerebral malaria, induced by the presence of a parasite, can pose this risk. Some bacteria, such as the staph that causes toxic shock syndrome, carry superantigens, which can cause an overwhelming immune response that can endanger a person's life. Suppressor cells are usually successful in keeping these effects from getting out of hand, but at times they fail, resulting in damage to the brain or other tissues such as those of the kidney. In addition to CD8 cells, a macrophage can also act as a suppressor cell by producing immunosuppressing factors when it recognizes that the immune response should be limited.

The Education of Lymphocytes

Long before they take part in an immune response, the cells of the immune system are born, mature, and are educated and trained to do their jobs. Most immune cells are born either in the thymus gland or in bone marrow. Those born in the bone marrow remain there until they mature or are sent to school in the thymus gland. Most immature T cells end up in the thymus gland for training.

The thymus is an endocrine gland located just over the heart. It is composed of two lobes that, together, are a little bigger than a man's fist. Here one of the great mysteries of the immune system takes place: cells are trained to differentiate self from nonself. They also select and develop receptor molecules so that they can recognize specific antigens. In this way, each immune cell develops its own identity and finds its life's work. The particular receptor gives it purpose. If a T cell is trained in the thymus to recognize a particular strain of meningitis or polio, it will react every time it encounters one of these viruses. It will be responsible for saving your life in the face of these disease-causing agents.

In keeping with the seriousness of its task, the thymus doesn't brook any form of incompetence. Ninety percent of the cells that go there for training never make it out alive. They self-destruct if they are unable to mature, to find a specific role in the overall immune armamentarium, or to learn to distinguish between self and nonself. Scientists don't understand exactly how this judgment is made and carried out, but we know it happens. Perhaps like weaker animals within herds, they are destroyed for the sake of the safety and health of the larger group. Clearly, behaviors that we see in nature that may shock us are also present within us. The immune system is dead serious about its mission, and the consequences for incompetence within its ranks are terminal.

Tolerance and Hypersensitivity

In almost all cases, the immune system does not attack the body itself and ignores harmless agents as well. This aspect of the system is referred to as tolerance. In effect, cells learn to ignore certain challenges. Tolerance gives the immune system the capacity to remain immobile in the face of certain antigens, including those produced by your own body and many harmless agents produced by our environment.

When the immune system loses such tolerance, it begins to

attack the body's own tissues. Called autoimmunity, this reaction to antigens occurs, for instance, in insulin-dependent diabetes (type I) in which the body destroys cells of the pancreas. This prevents the pancreas from creating insulin, a hormone that is essential to life. A similar chain of events characterizes rheumatoid arthritis, in which the immune system attacks the synovial tissues located in the joints. In these diseases, the immune system fails to differentiate self from nonself.

In other cases, the immune system reacts to harmless antigens, but in a way that damages the body. This form of hypersensitivity includes common allergies and dangerous immune reactions to drugs such as antibiotics. In the case of allergies, a harmless substance (such as ragweed pollen) triggers an immune reaction simply because the immune system does not recognize the pollen as harmless. In a sense, the immune system is out of focus; it can't see the fine details of the pollen and thus cannot discern the fact that this substance doesn't present a real threat.

Drugs can cause changes in the bloodstream that trigger an immune reaction. Penicillin and certain other sulfa drugs can bind with red blood cells, causing changes in the appearance of the red cells. In this case, the immune system perceives those red cells as foreign and attacks them — creating a dangerous condition. Other substances can bind with and change tissues and thus trigger an immune reaction. Pesticides, poison ivy, drugs, and even certain metal surfaces — such as the metal on the back of a watch — can sometimes effect changes in the cells and set off an immune reaction. In these so-called contact sensitivities, changes in the cells make the skin appear foreign to the immune system.

Still another example of intolerance involves transplanted organs and tissues donated from another person, which are often viciously attacked by immune cells. A heart transplant, for example, requires the use of powerful immunosuppressive drugs because the organ is seen as nonself by the immune system. In some cases, however, the donated organ is not attacked. That occurs when the organ's MHC molecule — the cuplike holder on the macrophage's cell membrane — is an identical match with the recipient of the organ. In this case, the MHC molecule is seen by the CD4 cells as normal, or self, and therefore dovetails smoothly with the overall immune defense system.

■ ■ ■

Even a passing familiarity with the intricacies of the immune system produces a sense of wonder. Indeed, our immune defenses often resemble the superheroes that our imaginations conjure up. And to make sure the system wins every battle, we now turn to the topic of immune system boosters — ways you can ensure the optimal functioning of your defense against disease.

CHAPTER THREE

How Immune System Boosters Work

Y OUR IMMUNE SYSTEM is powerful indeed, but like all living things, it requires the appropriate raw materials and a supportive environment to work at its best. By following a good diet and incorporating other immunity-boosting behaviors into your life, you can provide your system with many of the elements it needs to thrive.

In order to better understand the individual immune system boosters that follow, it's worth examining how certain behaviors weaken the immune system and contribute to disease. It's also important to understand, in general, how lifestyle can strengthen our defenses and help reestablish health.

Immune system boosters work in at least four general ways, which overlap somewhat with one another.

1. They enhance communication within the immune cell, which makes the actions of the cell more efficient and powerful.

2. They make immune cells more numerous, more aggressive, and more effective in the face of an antigen.

3. They significantly slow down, and in some cases halt, production of free radicals, the essential cause of more than sixty illnesses, including cancer, heart disease, brain disorders, and most of the symptoms of aging.

4. They have the long-term effect of significantly improving the environment within your blood and tissues where immune cells work, so that your immune system functions more optimally.

From a long-term perspective, immune system boosters are like capital that you place in a savings account, to be drawn on later when your immune system confronts an antagonist. By helping you maintain a healthy lifestyle, even when you are well, these boosters will make tomorrow's battles easier to win.

■ ■ ■

Though immune system boosters help your defenses work better, they are not what we typically think of as medicine. In modern orthodox health care, a medicine is thought of as an outside agent — a pill or potion — that defeats disease. We typically think of medicine as having an independent effect on an illness. These medications do not enlist the assistance of your body.

Immune system boosters, on the other hand, work by strengthening your body's own disease-fighting forces — not as substitutes for them. They can improve your health even in the short run and dramatically reduce your chances of becoming sick in the first place. Our immunity-boosting program helps prevent disease by building up the system that defeats challenges to your health each day.

Medicines, of course, are often essential to getting well, but some medicines depress the immune system. Antibiotics, for example, destroy bacteria independent of anything your body does. In effect, they work in place of your immune system, and possibly weaken it in the long run. Hence, the long-term use of medicines may leave your defenses weaker, whereas the long-term use of this program will strengthen your defenses and make you healthier. Throughout the book, we emphasize that each immune system booster works better in the company of the other boosters, rather than alone.

Tiny Factories

To visualize how immune system boosters work, think of immune cells as factories that manufacture various products. The nucleus of the cell can be seen as the corporate management team. Inside the cell, genes direct production of various products, such as cytokines (chemical messengers), antibodies, and an array of toxic chemicals that destroy bacteria, viruses, and cancer cells. Also, at times when demand increases, each factory expands to produce new factories, or cells — a process called mitosis. Like all factories, each cell needs raw materials in order to produce its products. These raw materials — carbohydrates, proteins, antioxidants, minerals, and other important nutrients — come mainly from your diet.

The Importance of Communication

Each cell manages a network of internal corporate communications. When an antigen is sensed by the antenna-like receptors on the outside of the cell, signals are passed from that receptor to the cell's nucleus. There the genes act according to these instructions. The receptors can be seen as the factory's marketing department — the workers who stay in touch with the outside world and its changing conditions.

The lines of communication must be open and working well in order for the cell to function properly. When the correct signals are passed from the receptors to the nucleus and then on to the genes, the cell responds appropriately to an antigen. In most cases, it is able to neutralize the antigen without creating the symptoms that alert you to the presence of a disease.

But if something interferes with the communication between the receptors and the nucleus, the immune cell may fail to function properly against an invader. The cell may respond only partially — that is, it may produce only small quantities of cytokines or chemical factors that destroy bacteria, viruses, or cancer cells. That weak response can allow the invader to multiply and gain a stronger foothold in the system. This happens very often among the elderly. Their immune systems can become weakened to the extent that they fail to produce normal levels of cytokines, such as tumor necrosis factor.

Another way the cell can backfire is to fail to reproduce in the face of a challenge. As we will show in Chapter 11, this sometimes happens when people suffer from bereavement due to the loss of a loved one. Lymphocytes simply fail to respond to a pathogen or a cancer cell. In other cases, the cell can literally self-destruct. This may benefit the system as a whole if food scarcity has made downsizing a priority; but sometimes the self-destruct message may go off by mistake, due to a breakdown in communication between the receptor and the nucleus. These problems reveal how important good communication is among the receptors, the nucleus, and the genes. And that communication is affected by the conditions in your blood and tissues, which, as we will see, are greatly influenced by your attitudes and daily behaviors.

The macrophages and the CD4 cells are most vulnerable to getting their signals crossed. Both depend upon the sensitivity of their receptors to determine exactly what type of antigen they are facing. Each cell must first recognize the type of antigen being encountered and then correctly pass on that information to its nucleus. As we pointed out in Chapter 2, only CD4 cells with the right receptor can respond to the specific type of antigen presented by the macrophage. The macrophage hopes that the CD4 cell with the right receptor will pass by and come in contact with the antigen. Once the CD4 cell with the correct receptor does this, it sends a set of signals to its nucleus, informing the nucleus of the presence of a particular type of challenge to the body.

That flow of information between the receptor and the nucleus — a series of delicate chemical reactions — can unfortunately be disrupted.

How the Flow of Information Becomes Blocked

The flow of information between receptor and nucleus can be disrupted by fat. When consumed in excess amounts, fat can coat and infiltrate the cell's receptor, much as the fat in milk coats a glass or the fat from steak coats a plate, and prevent it from recognizing antigens. Such infiltration upsets communication within the cell. Also, fat can clog the cell membrane, thus preventing macrophages from offering antigen to CD4 cells. Finally, dietary fat can prevent cytokine production from occurring in macrophages and CD4 cells. Both saturated fat, found in most animal foods, and polyunsaturated fats, found in vegetables and fish, can gum up CD4 cells and macrophages, if they are consumed in excess.

Studies have shown that women who eat excessive amounts of fish oils (a polyunsaturated fat that has been touted as a deterrent of heart disease) experience decreased production of cytokines, including interleukin-1, interleukin-2, and interleukin-6. You'll recall that interleukin-2 signals CD4 cells to replicate and thereby increases your immune response to a threatening agent. By diminishing the production of important interleukins, fats have widespread effects on all immune cells, including CD4 cells and B cells, and on antibody production. Thus, fats depress immune function.

Aging, Decay, and Free Radicals

Time takes its toll on all of us. We call it aging, but what really happens is a form of decay at the molecular level. Molecules are fairly stable until they come in contact with highly reactive oxygen molecules called oxidants. Oxidants have a degenerative effect on molecules, causing them to lose electrons, break up, and decay. As these molecules (called free radicals) fall apart, the cells and tissues do too. A free radical tries to gain back its lost electrons by stealing them from neighboring molecules, a destabilizing effect that can create scar tissue, cause inflammation and deformities, and break down cells' DNA, causing cancer. These decaying molecules cause most of the debilitating diseases we suffer from today, including cancer, heart disease, Alzheimer's, Parkinson's, cataracts, cirrhosis of the liver, and kidney disease. They also are responsible for most of the symptoms of aging that we're all too familiar with, including wasting of muscles, bone loss, and wrinkling of the skin.

Many factors can cause accelerated free radical production. Among the most common are x-rays, ultraviolet light, many forms of radiation, air pollution, ozone from car exhaust, sulfur dioxide (the main component of acid rain), drugs (both recreational and pharmaceutical), cigarette smoking, and fat — especially saturated fat — in our food. These free radical producers all contribute to aging and disease.

Your immune system must deal with free radicals. The rate at which your molecules decay determines both the burden upon your immune system and the speed with which you age. Fortunately, you have a lot of influence over how rapidly this happens. As we will see in the next chapter, one of the ways to slow free radical production and the aging process is to eat foods rich in the antioxidants — nutrients that stop the oxidation process and thereby slow the breakdown of your cells and tissues.

Immunity and the Mind

Particular behaviors also contribute to weakening the immune function or strengthening it. Your immune function is affected by the way you think, the emotions you feel, the stress you experience, and the quality of your relationships. These invisible influences are transformed into physical and chemical responses, including the production of hormones and brain chemicals called neurotransmitters. For example, stressful situations normally trigger the "fight or flight" response, in which biological and psychological conditioning spur you either to run from danger or to stand and fight it. Such stressful situations cause production of neurochemicals such as cortisol (a hormone that opens bronchial passageways, thus increasing respiration), enkephalins and endorphins (morphine-like compounds that diminish perception of pain), and adrenaline (a hormone that increases metabolism, respiration, and energy consumption).

The immune system responds to each of these chemicals. Cortisol, for example, binds with a specific receptor inside the CD4 cell. Once it attaches itself there, cortisol signals genes within the CD4 cell's nucleus to suppress production of important cytokines, such as interleukin-2 (IL-2). Since IL-2 promotes CD4 cell proliferation, cortisol keeps these T cells from multiplying and thereby depresses immune response. This is only one way that stress keeps you from having an optimal immune reaction when you encounter a virus or bacterium while under stress.

By the time we reach our fifties and sixties, we've experienced decades of stress and exposure to oxidants, which take their toll on the immune system. Consequently, aging is associated with depression of the immune function. Still, it isn't necessary to become resigned to this eventuality; research has shown that whenever immune system boosters are incorporated into people's lives — even late in life — the strength of the immune system returns.

Unfortunately, most of us do not give the system the support it needs to maintain optimal function. Hence, it weakens with age. And that weakening occurs in virtually every aspect of the immune system, especially in the CD4 cells. Studies have shown that CD4 cell function is markedly impaired with aging, in part because production of IL-2 drops significantly among the elderly. CD4 cells, or T cells, are not the only immune cells to suffer. Because of the accumulation of toxic stresses, B cells develop a variety of abnormalities and often fail to produce antibodies in sufficient quantities to deal effectively with foreign substances. They can, in fact, create autoantibodies, which attack the cells and tissues of the body. Granulocytes, too, become weakened with age.

These factors increase our susceptibility to degenerative illnesses. Meanwhile, the lifelong accumulation of injuries to DNA increases our chances of developing cancer. But as we said, immune system depression is avoidable. You can maintain the health and strength of your defenses by incorporating immune system boosters into your life.

Enter the Immune System Boosters

As you will see in the chapters that follow, there are many ways to promote immune response and even to restore its strength.

The first booster we'll discuss is the group of nutrients referred to as antioxidants. These compounds slow down and sometimes stop free radical production. They do this by donating electrons to decaying molecules and thereby stop the breakdown of molecules, cells, and tissues. They also improve communication within the cell, protect the cell's membrane, enhance the cell's ability to recognize antigens, and stimulate CD4 and natural killer cells to multiply in the face of an antigen.

Simply by reducing fat and cholesterol in your diet, you will improve the ability of your CD4 cells to respond appropriately to antigens. In addition, numerous minerals, herbs, specific nutrients, and behaviors can promote the health of individual im-

---

mune cells and overall immune function. Among the most effective immunity-boosting behaviors are moderate exercise, meditation, and relaxation techniques that utilize the power of the mind to support the body. Even the presence of supportive relationships in our lives plays a role in how well we fight disease.

■ ■ ■

All of the immune system boosters combine to encourage a health-promoting environment in the trenches — the blood and tissues where the immune wars are fought. Your tissues can be seen as a reserve from which your immune cells can draw antioxidants, minerals, and special nutrients when needed. Your immune system needs a whole range of nutrients in order to respond effectively to a challenging agent. In addition, it thrives in an environment that isn't polluted by harmful hormones or excess quantities of fat and cholesterol. Therefore, rather than focus exclusively on individual nutrients, we must also see the bigger picture, which is the need to provide a rich and healthy ecosystem within our tissues.

Hence, what you do in any given day matters less than what you do consistently over time. If you are eating healthful foods that include many immune system boosters, and if you're coping effectively with stress and maintaining a balanced life in terms of work and relationships, periodic deviations in lifestyle will not affect you very much. But if you're depriving your body of what it needs on an ongoing basis, you put yourself at risk.

■ ■ ■

But let's see how this information plays itself out in the life of Steve, a fictional human being. He will experience the immunity-depressing circumstances that many of us encounter each day. Fortunately, he's read about immune system boosters and has adopted an appropriate lifestyle. Here's how these boosters can make the difference between staying healthy or becoming seriously ill.

Steve's Immune System

Steve is a forty-year-old man of average health and fitness. He is married to Sally. Together they have two school-age children and a dog. Steve and Sally are interested in practical ways to improve their health and have made changes in lifestyle in order to protect themselves against disease. However, because most of what goes on inside of him is invisible to him, Steve doesn't know how powerful such changes really are at protecting him against illness. He is about to gain one of the more dramatic benefits from his improved lifestyle, though he will never know it.

Today, Steve will confront many of the typical substances that depress the immune system; in fact, most of us encounter these factors in a typical day. On top of this, he'll also be exposed to the tuberculosis bacterium (TB). While all of this is occurring, we'll track the events inside of Steve and see how his actions strengthen or depress his immune response in the face of an array of antagonists.

■ ■ ■

At the crack of dawn each weekday morning, Steve and his family wake up to a healthy breakfast, often oatmeal or a different cereal or grain, toast, and jam. Steve and his wife are both coffee drinkers. It is Monday, and the family is late and hurrying to their destinations: Steve and his wife, Sally, to their jobs; Heather and Kelly, the children, to their sixth- and fourth-grade classrooms. Unfortunately, the family ran out of cereal over the weekend, so instead, everyone eats toast and butter and throws down coffee or juice. The whole wheat bread is a good choice; the butter on the bread isn't. Also, Sally takes cream in her coffee; Steve drinks it black. Like the butter, cream is high in fat.

Fat, Free Radicals, and Steve's Immune System

Steve and his family start off the day with a small amount of butter, a free radical producer. Fortunately, the family members do not consume lots of fat, which reduces the impact of the fat on their immune systems. A small fraction of their macrophages may be temporarily dulled, but overall, blood cholesterol and triglycerides (fatty acids in the blood) are low. Therefore, the butter has little impact on their immune systems. Before they hurry out of the house, they take their brown-bag lunches out of the refrigerator and pass them around.

Air Pollution and Steve's Immune System

Steve and Sally get into their cars and leave for work; Steve drives the children to school on his way. Once he drops them off, he pulls onto the highway and joins the rush hour traffic. He lowers his window slightly and breathes in the air pollution — mostly from car exhaust composed primarily of carbon monoxide, ozone, cadmium, and other heavy metals, all of them free radical producers. Carbon monoxide lowers the blood's oxygen-carrying capacity, which will force the heart to work harder to bring oxygen to cells. Some cells will suffocate. Also, the toxic gas and other air pollutants will accumulate in tissue fluid, which will cause some damage to the immune system, making it less able to deal with viruses, bacteria, and other toxins that may be encountered during the day.

Thus Steve experiences another blow to his immune system on his way to work. And he meets this one on a daily basis.

Stress and an Unfortunate Encounter

Steve barely notices the drive to work. He's got deadlines approaching for various projects, all of which weigh heavily upon his mind. As he works out various scenarios — many of them with negative outcomes — his stress levels begin to rise.

Stress causes many changes in the body, including alterations in muscle behavior, respiration, hormone levels, and immune cell activity. But among the most common changes caused by stress is depression in natural killer cell activity and a reduction in the activity of T lymphocytes. Stress makes natural killer cells and T lymphocytes less active in the face of a pathogen. When healthy, these cells multiply rapidly when confronted by a challenge — such as a cancer cell, a virus, or a bacterium — and thus mount a more vigorous attack against any threat to the body. But under stress, especially chronic stress, natural killer cells and T lymphocytes do not multiply as rapidly, and in extreme conditions, may even remain dormant when presented with an antigen.

As if pollution and stress were not enough of a challenge, Steve is cut off by another car that veers wildly into Steve's lane, as the other driver exits the highway. Steve's anger triggers another explosion of chemical events within his body. Heart rate and blood pressure skyrocket. His adrenal glands pump adrenaline; respiration increases; the liver secretes glycogen into the bloodstream to increase energy reserves. Fat cells release their contents into the bloodstream as a result of that adrenaline rush; although this makes more energy available, its overall effect is to tax the immune system further by forcing macrophages to gobble up those fat particles. The stress also causes a direct impact on the immune cells.

Unless Steve is an accomplished Zen monk, these reactions are unavoidable; stress and anger are normal reactions to demanding and threatening situations. Thus, by the time Steve pulls into the parking lot of his workplace, his immune system has been weakened somewhat.

Steve hurries into the building and runs toward elevator doors that are closing. A helpful person stops the doors, and Steve slides into the crowded elevator. "Thanks," he says to the person who held the doors. The words are no sooner out of his mouth than a person standing to his side sneezes directly into Steve's face. Unfortunately, the person is a tuberculosis carrier.

Involuntarily, Steve breathes in. He doesn't know it, but he has been exposed to TB.

A Little about TB

Each year, *Mycobacterium tuberculosis* — the bacterium that causes tuberculosis — causes 8 million new cases of TB and kills 2.9 million people worldwide. Between 1881 and 1985, the disease was in retreat, largely because of improved sanitation and more vigorous methods of treatment. In the early part of this century, antibiotics emerged that could destroy the bacterium. For the next fifty years, the numbers of people who died from the disease steadily decreased. However, since 1985, the pattern has reversed itself, and the numbers of people who contract TB have gone up steadily.

Several reasons explain TB's resurgence, but among the most important is the spread of AIDS (acquired immune deficiency syndrome). AIDS attacks and weakens the human immune system and consequently makes it more vulnerable to other infectious diseases, including TB. This increased population of carriers serves as a source of infection for those with whom they come in contact.

TB bacteria are carried on water particles in the air or even on simple dust particles. Because it is airborne, TB is easily communicated among people, unlike HIV. A person with the illness can spread it to others by sneezing, coughing, or even speaking. It can also be transmitted when dust particles are raised by moving air and breathed into the lungs by an unsuspecting person. TB, of course, can be life threatening.

But TB is much more likely to take hold within a body guarded by a weakened immune system. Ninety percent of those who encounter TB do not manifest symptoms because, once inhaled, the bacteria are destroyed by a healthy immune system. In most cases, immune cells recognize the bacteria immediately and destroy them in the lungs. Even a person kissed by someone with TB usually avoids the illness because the gastric juices in the stomach destroy the bacteria before they have a chance to make their way into the bloodstream. The bacterium is killed by sunlight, as well. Therefore, rooms well lit with sunlight are usually free of the TB organism.

TB is reaching epidemic proportions also because the bacteria have become increasingly resistant to standard antibiotics. Drug resistance has emerged largely because infected people have often stopped treatment before the bacteria are fully destroyed, which has given the TB time to adapt to the antibiotics. Thus, while TB has become more resistant to medical therapy, the human immune system — collectively speaking — appears to be getting weaker. These factors combine to give TB a stronger foothold everywhere.

TB has reached epidemic proportions in the United States. Moreover, until new drugs are created, multi-drug-resistant TB can be combated only by strong immune systems — just one more reason why we must take better care of ourselves.

Back at the Office

Once in his office, Steve drinks more coffee and thus keeps his adrenaline levels high. At this moment, things don't look good for Steve, but he's about to start turning things around.

Unlike the trip in the car, when his mind was focused on the dark side of his pressing issues, Steve can attack his problems and use his competence to gain control over a challenging situation. He now sets to work. The research shows that Steve can do a great deal to boost his immune function throughout the rest of his day. He does not have to be victimized by difficulties. Rather, he can fight back.

First, Steve delegates various tasks and asks his coworkers for help with his pressing deadlines. This immediately disperses some of the pressure and relieves stress. He begins to feel supported and connected to the larger workplace community. Such feelings of connectedness and support relieve stress and boost immunity. Relief of stress causes T lymphocytes and macrophages to be less sluggish and more responsive to challenges to the system, including bacterial invaders such as TB.

In addition to the sense of support, Steve feels more control over his environment and the source of his stress. This has a major impact on his sense of well-being and his immune system. Animal studies and a few human studies have shown significant diminution of immune system function and increased susceptibility to infections in subjects who are under chronic stress. However, when both laboratory animals and humans experience a sense of control over stressful situations or see adversity as a challenge, the ill effects of stress become neutralized. Natural killer cells and T lymphocytes are directly affected for the better.

Because Steve doesn't surrender to his problems, his efforts pay off in a heightened immune response. Studies have found that women diagnosed with cancer who faced it with a fighting spirit had greater survival rates after both five years and ten years than did those who felt helpless or who stoically accepted their cancer. The likely reason is greater immune response in the face of a challenge.

By lunchtime, Steve is gaining momentum, and the brown-bag lunch he's brought with him is his ace in the hole. He brought brown rice with some sunflower seeds sprinkled on top, a cup of cooked collard greens mixed with balsamic vinegar, leftover potatoes, an orange, and an apple.

Antioxidants and Steve's Immune System

Steve's lunch contains a bounty of nutrients that will boost his immune system. And among the most powerful of those boosters are compounds in foods called antioxidants. They help prevent the devastating effect on health that free radicals cause. Antioxidants donate electrons to atoms, cells, and tissues, and thereby stabilize or halt decay. Also called free radical scavengers, they promote immune cell activity as well.

The three most familiar antioxidants are vitamins C and E and beta-carotene, the vegetable source of vitamin A. Selenium, vitamin B_6, and glutathione are also important. Steve's lunch is rich in all of these antioxidants. First, the brown rice and seeds are good sources of vitamin E and glutathione. Both are powerful free radical scavengers, and both boost cellular immune function. The collard greens and the orange provide vitamin C, one of the most powerful antioxidants and immune system boosters in the food supply. It is particularly protective against heart disease because it prevents cholesterol from decaying and eventually forming atherosclerotic plaques. The leafy greens and the apple in Steve's lunch contain plenty of beta-carotene, which stops the breakdown of cells and tissues caused by free radical formation. It increases the number of several kinds of immune cells and makes them more potent against disease, including cancer cells. Finally, the brown rice and seeds are good sources of zinc, a mineral that powerfully boosts the immune system. Zinc wards off all forms of infection and promotes B cells, which produce antibodies that attack antigens.

Steve's lunch contains other nutrients — complex carbohydrates for energy, fiber for healthy digestion — which positively influence his overall health. Moreover, Steve consumes generous portions of these nutrients, which means the effect on his health will be significant.

Also important, this type of lunch — composed of grains, vegetables, and fruit — is customary for Steve. On the days that he doesn't bring his lunch, he stops at a local restaurant for a sandwich on whole grain bread, a salad, and steamed fresh vegetables; he also buys a piece of fruit from a street vendor. Steve has discovered what many Americans have known for some time: healthful food is a lot easier to get than many people believe. At a Chinese restaurant, he can get brown rice, steamed vegetables, and oranges. At fast food joints, he can get a large salad and a whole wheat bun, on which he puts his salad to make a green sandwich. He also gets a carton of orange juice and an apple. At a nearby Japanese restaurant, Steve gets miso soup (which contains a phytochemical called genistein that research has shown stops the growth of tumors — more on genistein later in the book), rice, vegetables, noodles, and other healthful dishes. Steve loves Italian food, especially pasta and marinara sauce, a dish that is low in fat and rich in vitamin C and other nutrients. With his meal, he gets a green salad loaded with antioxidants and fiber. There are a lot of choices, Steve has learned, and he's continually coming up with new ideas. Hence, Steve builds his reserves of important vitamins and minerals on a daily basis.

A Little Exercise Booster

Following his lunch, Steve takes a quick walk around the block. He thinks of it as simply working off some steam and getting a second wind, but it too strengthens his immune system. Studies have shown that moderate exercise improves the ability of macrophages to neutralize viruses and bacteria. Like so many other immune system boosters Steve has employed today, the little walk enhances the performance of macrophages and thus targets the TB he inhaled this morning.

Steve works hard and productively for the next couple of hours, but at 3:00 P.M., he hits the wall. He's a little stiff and a little tired, and his eyes get heavy. He hasn't scheduled any pressing meetings, so he decides to take another quick walk to get his circulation going. After the walk, he munches on the uneaten apple from his lunch and feels refreshed. The apple contains another round of beta-carotene and plenty of fiber, which lowers his cholesterol and diminishes ever so slightly the burden on his macrophages. By the time he has finished work, he's had a full day of boosting his immune system.

Dinner and More Immune System Boosters

On the drive home, Steve feels accomplished and optimistic — this attitude helps macrophages, T lymphocytes, and natural killer cells function smoothly. He pops a tape into the car stereo and listens to music, another immunity enhancer. The music encourages a relaxation response, which releases muscle tension and reduces stress.

At home, Steve and Sally prepare a delicious dinner, which contains a variety of powerful immune system boosters. The main dish is white fish with a simple orange sauce, cooked with a variety of mild spices, including cumin. A baked potato and a vegetable medley that includes kale, carrots, and shiitake mushrooms, sautéed in a light sesame oil and garlic sauce, round out the meal. Finally, there's a salad with an olive oil and balsamic vinegar dressing.

While he cooks, Steve drinks a beer, which he does routinely after work. However, because Steve drinks in moderation — one beer or glass of red wine daily on average — the alcohol has little or no effect on his immune system. In fact, some studies suggest that in moderate quantity it may promote production of HDL (high-density lipoprotein) cholesterol — the good cholesterol — and have a mild boosting effect on the immune system.

The family meal, on the other hand, borders on being downright medicinal. To begin with, it is low in fat, especially saturated fat, which itself takes stress off the immune system. It is loaded with antioxidants and minerals. It also includes herbs and other ingredients, especially shiitake mushrooms and garlic, that enhance the immune system's performance.

Research has established the shiitake mushroom as an impressive cancer fighter and a powerful cholesterol-lowering food. Its antiviral and antibacterial properties encourage Steve's immune system to fight against the TB. Garlic has also been shown to enhance health in many ways. It stimulates lymphocytes and macrophages to respond more vigorously to an antigen, and it prompts the liver to metabolize and neutralize carcinogens that would otherwise produce cancer cells and tumors.

After dinner, Sally has a cup of chamomile tea, an herbal tea that has been shown to encourage macrophages to consume (or phagocytize) bacteria and viruses.

Numerous intangibles in Steve's life promote a stronger immune response. Steve has a loving intimacy with his wife and children. Such close relationships benefit the immune system. They have been shown to promote longevity, particularly among people struggling against a life-threatening disease. Steve also keeps fairly consistent hours. He gets up at the same time each day and goes to bed at about the same time. This, too, is a health-supporting habit.

Finally, he gets a good night's sleep, the last immune system booster of the day. The body requires a certain amount of rest, particularly deep sleep, in order to maintain a healthy immune function. During deep sleep, the body slows down many of its activities so that it can focus its energies and immune defenses on healing.

Three Months Later

Tuberculosis requires two to eight weeks to manifest symptoms and be diagnosed. Three months after encountering the bacteria, Steve is fine. He has no symptoms of illness. His immune system has emerged victorious over the TB that Steve doesn't even know he encountered.

PART II

The Ten Best Immune System Boosters

CHAPTER FOUR

Immune System Booster #1:
The Antioxidants

THERE IS PROBABLY NO more celebrated group of nutrients in the food supply today than the antioxidants. They prevent disease, boost the immune system, and even slow the aging process. In fact, they may be the most powerful health enhancers in the food supply.

Nevertheless, much is misunderstood about these essential nutrients. First, you do not have to purchase expensive pills to be healthy. In fact, recent studies have shown that getting the antioxidant beta-carotene in pill form may even increase the risk of disease for some people, a finding that has created enormous confusion. Many people wonder if antioxidants aren't all that they were cracked up to be; others worry that they may be just a little dangerous. Antioxidants are in fact essential to good health, but the way in which you get them is as important as the nutrients themselves. For the most part, antioxidants are most effective when you get them in the old-fashioned way: as part of the food you eat.

Antioxidants appear to be more effective when they work in combination with other immunity-boosting, cancer-fighting nutrients that are also present in food. This certainly appears to be the case with beta-carotene, a nutrient that, when eaten as food, is clearly an important immune system booster. Taken in pill form, it doesn't seem to have the same effectiveness, and there is even a slight chance of its raising the risk of cancer among cigarette smokers; why this occurs is still unknown.

The only antioxidant that may be worth supplementing to your healthy diet is vitamin E. Supplements of two hundred milligrams per day or more appear to have a positive effect on immune response, without any evidence of harmful side effects.

Even if you decide to take additional vitamin E, don't rely entirely on the supplements. The best way to get your antioxidants is to eat plenty of apples, oranges, leafy greens, broccoli, cantaloupe, brown rice, olive oil, and many other delicious foods. These whole grains, vegetables, and fruits contain an abundance of antioxidants, as well as other cancer fighters and immune system boosters. Simply by eating these and other foods, you can protect yourself from allergies, arthritis, the common cold, the flu, cataracts, cancer, and heart disease, just to name a handful of illnesses. In many instances, these potent allies can help you overcome chronic and serious illnesses, as well as keep you younger and fitter.

Treating the Cause of Illness and Aging: Oxidation

Antioxidants attack the very causes of illness, depression of the immune system, and aging. The most common diseases today occur because cells, tissues, and organs break down, or decay, through oxidation (discussed in detail in Chapter 3). Oxidation creates free radicals, destabilized molecules that form scar tissue at very sensitive locations throughout your body, including your skin, arteries, eyes, and brain. Damaged tissue replaces normal tissue but can't fulfill its normal function. When scar tissue manifests itself in the collagen of your skin, you get wrinkles; when it manifests itself in your eyes, you can contract cataracts; when it manifests itself in your brain, you can suffer Alzheimer's or Parkinson's diseases.

Scar tissue isn't the only problem caused by free radicals, however. They arise in your bloodstream to form cholesterol plaque in your arteries that can lead to heart attacks and strokes. They cause inflammation in your joints and deformities in your bones, resulting in arthritis. Free radicals also can weaken and impair the immune system. Most dangerous of all, they can break down your cells' DNA and cause cancer. In all, free radicals are responsible for more than sixty major illnesses — the very diseases that deform, disable, and kill most of us today.

Oxidants: Those You Can Avoid and Those You Cannot

It would be nice if we could avoid oxidants and free radicals, but we can't. Many free radicals are formed because your cells produce oxidants in the normal course of their work. Simply by utilizing oxygen and nutrition to rebuild the body, cells produce oxidants, which in turn create free radicals. Mammals — including humans — tend to produce oxidants at very different speeds, depending on how fast their metabolisms work. According to researcher Bruce N. Ames, Ph.D., and his colleagues at the University of California, Berkeley, the DNA in each of your cells receives approximately ten thousand hits per day from oxidants, a lot of injuries to the command centers of your cells. Such attacks can injure your DNA, either disabling and killing the cell or creating mutations, including possible cancers. Fortunately, the nucleus of each cell, in which the DNA is stored, has enzymes that repair the DNA and heal most of these injuries. But some injuries remain unrepaired and can eventually cause cancer.

So far, we've spoken mainly about the oxidants that occur through normal metabolism, but most of the oxidants that attack your cells don't come from your normal metabolic processes but from poisons you take into your body. Air pollution, cigarette smoke, dietary fat and cholesterol, radiation (including excessive exposure to sunlight), alcohol, recreational and pharmaceutical drugs, and chemical pollutants are the major sources of oxidants and free radicals that your body must combat every day. A great many of these are avoidable, which means that your behavior dictates to a great extent how rapidly you will age, how quickly you will become ill, and whether or not you will have to deal with a particular disease at all.

Stopping Free Radicals in Their Tracks

This is where *antioxidants* come into the picture. Also known as free radical scavengers, antioxidants restore stability to molecules, cells, and tissues by donating electrons to decaying molecules. They prevent the need for molecules to steal electrons from their neighbors. In this way, antioxidants slow and in many cases stop the oxidative process, which is one way they prevent disease and slow aging. As we said in Chapter 1, research is now showing that antioxidants may be able to reduce the incidence of certain common degenerative diseases by half.

In addition to the familiar vitamins C and E and beta-carotene, antioxidants include vitamin B_6, glutathione, bioflavonoids (a group of compounds found in vegetable foods), several minerals (including selenium, zinc, copper, and manganese), and an amino acid called L-cysteine.

In order to get adequate quantities of antioxidants, *you should eat at least five servings of whole grains, vegetables, and fruits per day, in almost any combination.* People who do not eat at least those five servings each day are at increased risk of illness, and this includes the vast majority of Americans. Dr. Ames and his colleagues have calculated that those who fail to eat the recommended five servings of antioxidant-rich foods have twice the risk of developing cancer as those who do. The elderly are particularly at risk because they often fail to get an adequate supply of antioxidants in their diets. However, when senior citizens increase their intake of antioxidants, their immune systems rebound to normal strength. In fact, the same happens for people in all age groups.

The Major Antioxidants

In the following pages, we will examine the effects of the most potent antioxidants on the immune system. We will also report how antioxidants prevent disease and may even be effective in the treatment of certain illnesses.

Beta-Carotene

Beta-Carotene and the Immune System

Your body uses beta-carotene to synthesize, or create, vitamin A, which is why beta-carotene is often referred to as the vegetable source of vitamin A. Beta-carotene is one member of a family consisting of hundreds of nutrients collectively called *carotenoids*. They are found in all colored vegetables and fruits, such as collard greens, kale, mustard greens, dark lettuce (such as romaine), broccoli, pumpkin, squash, carrots and other root vegetables, brussels sprouts, and virtually all colorful fruit, such as apples, pears, strawberries, blueberries, blackberries, and cherries. You get tens of carotenoids — sometimes even hundreds — whenever you eat a green, orange, or yellow vegetable. This, of course, is yet another argument for eating a wide variety of vegetables.

The way most carotenoids affect health remains a mystery to science simply because they have not yet been studied closely. Many of them, if not all, could be immune system boosters and cancer fighters; we don't yet know. Beta-carotene, however, has been studied, and the research makes it look pretty good.

To begin with, beta-carotene stops the breakdown of cells and tissues caused by oxidation and free radical formation. In the process, it takes the stress off your immune system and slows the speed at which you age. In addition, beta-carotene appears to increase the number of several types of immune cells, including

CD4 cells and natural killer cells, whenever your body confronts some form of disease. It also makes these cells stronger against infection, cancer, and heart disease.

Beta-carotene has been shown to strengthen the immune system's effort against *Candida albicans,* the most common cause of yeast infections. Vitamin A has been shown to dramatically reduce infections, particularly those of the intestinal tract and lungs. It also greatly reduces the number of deaths due to infections in children with vitamin A deficiency.

Beta-Carotene and Heart Disease

Numerous studies have shown that beta-carotene is particularly effective in preventing fat and cholesterol from being oxidized and forming atherosclerosis, the cholesterol plaque that causes heart attacks and strokes. Its effectiveness at slowing oxidation of fats has led researchers to suggest that beta-carotene also may be a potent form of therapy for heart disease patients.

Women who ate five or more servings of carrots per week had 68 percent fewer strokes than those who ate carrots only once a month. Other studies have shown a reduction in the number of heart attacks among those whose diets included similar amounts of foods rich in beta-carotene.

Beta-Carotene and Cancer

Beta-carotene has also been suggested to protect the body against cancer. The nutrient stimulates macrophages to produce tumor necrosis factor, a cancer-killing chemical capable of destroying cancer cells.

A study published in the medical journal *Cancer* (March 15, 1991) demonstrated that beta-carotene supplementation in men with cancer — either of the mouth or the esophagus — increased the percentage of T cells and natural killer cells. The researchers found that the beta-carotene significantly improved the ability of natural killer cells to kill cancer cells.

A large population study of sixty-five hundred Chinese done by Cornell researchers found that daily consumption of foods high in beta-carotene was associated with low rates of certain cancers, particularly stomach cancer.

However, recent studies have cast doubt on whether it is the beta-carotene in foods that is protective or other carotenoids found in the same foods. In these studies, supplements of beta-carotene did not protect against cancer.

Vitamin C

Vitamin C and the Immune System

Vitamin C may be the most effective antioxidant available in the food supply, according to scientists at University of California at Berkeley, because of its remarkable ability to reduce the amount of oxidation taking place within cells. At the same time, vitamin C causes the immune system to respond more vigorously to viruses, bacteria, and cancer cells. It also prevents the inflammation produced by a vigorous immune response, thus reducing the discomfort that normally accompanies colds and infection.

Vitamin C and Heart Disease

Because of its powerful antioxidant properties, vitamin C prevents the oxidation of fats that leads to atherosclerosis, heart attacks, and strokes. Some recent studies suggest that vitamin C may be even more protective than vitamin E against atherosclerosis, which has been celebrated in the popular press for its protection against heart disease. In one study that compared the effects of vitamin C to those of vitamin E, researchers discovered that *oxidation of lipids was stopped entirely* while vitamin C was present in the bloodstreams of those being studied.

A study done at the Harvard School of Public Health found that vitamin C prevents LDL (low-density lipoprotein — the "bad cholesterol") particles from being oxidized, by surrounding the LDL particle with a protective coating. Other research has found that people over the age of sixty who eat at least 180 milligrams of vitamin C per day — an amount you can obtain in a couple of stalks of broccoli — had 11 percent higher HDL cholesterol (the good kind that prevents heart disease) and had half the risk of contracting high blood pressure than those who did not eat at least that much vitamin C per day.

At UCLA, a study of more than eleven thousand men found that those whose diets were rich in vitamin C had a 45 percent lower death rate from heart disease than men whose diets were low in vitamin C.

Vitamin C and Cancer

Epidemiological research has shown that people whose diets are richer in vitamin C than those whose are deficient have lower rates of breast, colon, rectal, and prostate cancers.

Recommended Doses of Vitamin C

Excessive intake of vitamin C (tolerance varies among individuals) can cause gastric and urinary tract disorders. Optimal amounts, even for elderly people who are often deficient in vitamin C, appears to be 100 milligrams per day. Research published in the *Journal of Age and Aging* (May 1991) revealed that 100 milligrams brought blood levels back to normal and, when combined with vitamin E and beta-carotene, positively affected all immune parameters tested. One can easily reach these blood levels by daily intake of foods rich in vitamin C. One spear of broccoli, for example, contains 134 milligrams of vitamin C.

Vitamin E

Vitamin E and the Immune System

Also known as tocopherol, vitamin E is essential to the maintenance of normal metabolism and healthy immune system functioning. The vitamin is especially protective against the normal age-related decline of the immune system. It reduces muscle damage, including the breakdown of muscle cells after exercise.

Those who do not get enough vitamin E, on average, suffer from a weakened immune response and more infectious diseases. However, by increasing intake of vitamin E, the immune response is boosted significantly. CD4 cells and granulocytes respond more vigorously to the presence of disease. Natural killer cells are stimulated to seek out and destroy viruses and cancer cells. Immune cells communicate among themselves better because of an increase in production of certain cytokines.

Not only does vitamin E cause a short-term improvement of immune function, but also research has shown that people who supplemented their diets with two hundred milligrams of vitamin E per day for six months experienced sustained and dramatic improvement of their immune response.

"After a person takes supplements of vitamin E, the immune system responds more vigorously to antigens," says Mohsen Meydani, Ph.D., associate professor of nutrition at the Antioxidant Research Laboratory at Tufts University. "Overall immune response is strengthened by vitamin E, because it spurs immune cells to multiply more rapidly in the presence of an antigen."

Vitamin E and Cancer

Vitamin E is associated with a lower incidence of cancer, especially cancer of the stomach, when it is consumed in quantities that double the ten-milligram dose given in the recommended daily allowance (RDA).

Vitamin E and Heart Disease

In a huge study of 87,245 nurses, vitamin E intake was shown to cut in half the risk of heart attack. Vitamin E protects against coronary heart disease by preventing LDL cholesterol from being oxidized, or changed into atherosclerotic plaques. At least one study found that low blood levels of vitamin E was the single most important predictor of death from heart disease — even more predictive than blood cholesterol levels. Vitamin E also lowers blood cholesterol and thus protects against the formation of cholesterol plaque; remarkably, vitamin E intake has been shown to reduce the actual size of the plaques in the arteries.

Recommended Doses of Vitamin E

Vitamin E may be the only antioxidant that is worth supplementing, if one's diet does not include ample amounts of whole grains and vegetables. On the other hand, long-term consumption of whole grains and fresh vegetables is associated with high blood levels of vitamin E and protection against degenerative illnesses. Still, many scientists are arguing for supplementation because research shows that the effects of vitamin E are particularly powerful above sixty milligrams per day. Most people can get thirty milligrams per day by eating grains, seeds, and vegetable oils. Dr. Meydani and others point out that when vitamin E is consumed consistently over time, even small amounts seem to boost the immune system. However, if blood levels of vitamin E are low, a supplement may be helpful until the overall diet is improved. If you take a vitamin E supplement, small doses are recommended — sixty to one hundred milligrams is the mostly widely recommended amount.

Vitamin B₆

Vitamin B_6 is an antioxidant and an essential nutrient in the production of cytokines, such as interleukin-2. When the supply of B_6 is inadequate, lymphocyte proliferation is significantly diminished. Deficiencies of B_6 are especially common among gay men infected with HIV; such deficiencies are due primarily to inadequate intake of foods containing B_6.

Lymphocyte proliferation is boosted when foods rich in B_6 are consumed.

Bioflavonoids

Bioflavonoids help to protect us against environmental poisons, such as automobile exhaust, dioxin, industrial effluents, and air pollutants. All of these contain toxins, collectively called aromatic hydrocarbons, which bind to receptors of cells. Once they are attached to the receptor, they are transported to the nucleus where they can damage DNA, causing mutations and cancer.

Bioflavonoids bind to the same receptors on the cells that would otherwise take up the chemical pollutants. Since this binding is competitive — there are only so many receptors and therefore it's a first come, first served arrangement — the bioflavonoids prevent the uptake of the chemical pollutants, thus protecting the cell's nucleus from these poisons.

Bioflavonoids have also been shown to prevent oxidation of LDL cholesterol and reduce the tendency of platelets to form clots, or thrombi, inside of arteries, which are responsible for most heart attacks. A study from the Netherlands shows fewer strokes in people who consume the most bioflavonoids.

Synergistic Effects

No single nutrient is a panacea. Nutrients work in harmony with one another. Often the effectiveness of one nutrient depends on the presence of another. For example, vitamin C has been found to help regenerate vitamin E. A lack of vitamin C results in lower levels of vitamin E in the bloodstream. Some studies suggest that vitamin C may play a protective role for other antioxidants as well. Perhaps vitamin C is such a powerful antioxidant that it neutralizes the greatest sources of oxidants, thus preserving high levels of other antioxidants.

When taken together, vitamins A, C, and E significantly boost immunity, especially among the elderly. Increased intake of antioxidants has been shown to significantly improve the morbidity and mortality rates of undernourished elderly people. In addition, all three major antioxidants combine to enhance the ratio between CD4 cells and the CD8 suppressor cells.

There is a growing belief among researchers that the consumption of antioxidants — especially the big three, beta-carotene and vitamins C and E — should be used as a therapy for AIDS patients.

Antioxidants and Other Illnesses

The preceding information was based on research that examined individual antioxidants, such as beta-carotene, or vitamins C and E. The following section examines the relationship between antioxidant consumption and specific disorders.

Arthritis

Low levels of antioxidants in the blood increase the risk of developing rheumatoid arthritis and heighten the severity of the disease for those who already have it. A study of 1,419 Finnish men and women followed for over twenty years showed that those with the lowest blood levels of antioxidants were eight times more likely to develop rheumatoid arthritis than those with the highest levels.

Many people report improvements in symptoms of arthritis

after taking beta-carotene, vitamin C, vitamin E, and selenium (a mineral antioxidant). Andrew Weil, M.D., has reported prescribing an antioxidant formula of beta-carotene, vitamins C and E, selenium, vitamin B₆, and the herb feverfew *(Tanacetum parthenium),* which has produced positive results for his patients. (See Chapter 7 for more on herbs.)

In several studies, patients taking from one hundred to six hundred milligrams of vitamin E per day have experienced significant pain relief and a reduction of inflammation from arthritis. It is also interesting that aurofin, a gold compound frequently used to treat rheumatoid arthritis, acts as a free radical scavenger.

Asthma

Asthma generates oxidants, which contribute to the severity of the disease. In one small study, patients showed improvement of their symptoms after taking nine hundred milligrams per day of vitamin E for several months. Several studies suggest that antioxidants in general reduce the severity of asthma and perhaps should be used in its treatment.

Cancer

Oxidation and free radical formation combine to cause cancer by disrupting the cells' DNA, making them mutate and reproduce themselves continuously. Certain sources of oxidants and free radicals are particularly effective at producing cancer, such as cigarette smoking, fat consumption, and exposure to ultraviolet light.

These cancer threats are reduced when antioxidants are consumed in regular and optimal amounts.

Cataracts

Cataracts are caused when cells and tissues in the lens of the eye are oxidized, causing opaque scar tissue to form that can result in partial or complete loss of sight. Antioxidants in general and vitamin E in particular appear to offer significant protection against cataract formation. However, it is important to combine a diet rich in antioxidants with the avoidance of substances that raise the level of oxidants in your bloodstream, such as cigarette smoke and high-fat foods. Cataracts may seem relatively minor compared to many other illnesses, but the disease is so prevalent that it accounts for the single largest Medicare expenditure.

Infection

Studies have shown that antioxidants significantly reduce the number and severity of infections, including the common cold.

Multiple Sclerosis

Although the findings are very preliminary, two animal studies have shown that a retinoic acid compound, a form of vitamin A, reduces the severity of both the acute and chronic (relapsing) forms of multiple sclerosis.

Optimal Amounts and Where You Can Get Them

Antioxidants are concentrated in whole grains, fresh vegetables, beans, fruit, and vegetable oils. Most grains, vegetables, and fruits contain multiple antioxidants, meaning that if you eat a leafy green vegetable, you're going to get vitamin C, vitamin E, beta-carotene, and perhaps dozens of other carotenoids. At the end of this chapter is a list of the major antioxidants, their primary sources, and how much you need to consume of them each day.

There is considerable debate today over whether or not we should take supplements of antioxidants and other nutrients that boost the immune system. Food contains so many immunity-boosting and cancer-fighting nutrients that no amount of supple-ments — no matter how many pills you take — could equal the value of whole grains, vegetables, fruits, seeds, and nuts.

The study of nutrition's effect on the immune system continues. Many nutrients are only now being discovered, such as the phytoestrogens and bioflavonoids, that fight cancer and boost the immune system. Others may yet be discovered and may ultimately prove essential to good health.

Relationships between nutrients present another new field of study. Clearly, the antioxidants work better together than they do alone. Subtle relationships exist between, say, vitamin C and E, or vitamin E and beta-carotene, that are only now being discovered. Much is unknown about how nutrients interact or strengthen each other's effects on the body.

Nutritious food, of course, benefits not only the immune system, but also the functioning of the entire body. A good example is fiber — a constituent of food that lowers blood levels of fat, cholesterol, and estrogen, while improving intestinal function and health. When you eat brown rice or collard greens or a carrot or an apple, you are getting a variety of antioxidants and other immune system boosters; you are also eating a plethora of health-enhancing and cancer-fighting nutrients, such as minerals, complex carbohydrates, proteins, and fiber. In other words, whole foods provide an array of health-promoting factors that may not have a direct impact on immunity, yet are essential to good health. All authorities agree that there is no substitute for a good diet, even when supplementation is called for.

Nevertheless, sometimes supplementation may be a wise choice. These cases include the elderly, especially men and women who have had long histories with poor diets and now have trouble tolerating the high fiber that accompanies a healthy diet. The best advice for people in this category is to improve the diet gradually, while taking an array of low-dose vitamins and mineral supplements. High doses can be toxic, as well as expensive and unnecessary — there is little or no evidence that a high dose of any nutrient, with the possible exception of vitamin E, provides any significant benefit to immune response.

Men and women infected with HIV may also benefit from

supplements. Supplementation may boost immunity among people with immune disorders, especially for those with a deficiency of one or more nutrients. A simple blood test can tell you if you are deficient in essential nutrients.

Finally, small children who resist eating a healthy diet may require supplements. Once again, there is no substitute for healthy foods — and no supplement will entirely offset the toxic effects of a poor diet — but a multivitamin and multimineral supplement will provide essential nutrients that the diet may lack and thereby maintain a healthy immune function.

If You Supplement, Keep Doses Small

If you decide to take a supplement, small amounts are better than the larger doses. Research published in *The Lancet* (November 11, 1992) demonstrated the effects of adding certain key nutrients to the diets of ninety-six senior citizens, all of whom were sixty-six years old and older. The seniors were divided into two groups, one of which was given a placebo (a pill containing some calcium and magnesium), while the experimental group was given supplements containing the following nutrients:

- Beta-carotene (16 milligrams)
- Calcium (200 milligrams)
- Copper (1.4 milligrams)
- Folate (400 micrograms)
- Iodine (0.2 milligrams)
- Iron (16 milligrams)
- Magnesium (100 milligrams)
- Niacin (16 milligrams)
- Riboflavin (1.5 milligrams)
- Selenium (20 micrograms)
- Thiamine (2.2 milligrams)

- Vitamin A (120 micrograms)
- Vitamin B_6 (3 milligrams)
- Vitamin B_{12} (4 micrograms)
- Vitamin C (80 milligrams)
- Vitamin D (4 micrograms)
- Vitamin E (44 milligrams)
- Zinc (14 milligrams)

Both groups were followed for one year. The researchers found that the supplemented group had significantly fewer infections and sick days; the supplemented group suffered a total of twenty-three sick days, compared to forty-eight sick days recorded by the placebo group. Blood tests revealed that the supplemented group had stronger immune responses and a greater number of circulating macrophages and other immune cells.

Moreover, these benefits were accomplished on relatively small doses of nutrient supplementation. As the researchers point out, "It is important to note that large-dose supplements were not used; indeed, very large doses of many micronutrients may impair immunity."

■ ■ ■

The following list of foods containing antioxidants shows clearly that these compounds are concentrated primarily in whole grains, fresh vegetables, beans, and fruit. The U.S. Surgeon General and other leading health authorities recommend a diet rich in these foods. If these foods make up the center of your diet, you will get an abundance of antioxidants and nutrients that will boost your immune system.

Much of the information on the nutritional content of foods is based on "The Diet Balancer" (Nutridata Software Corporation, Wappinger Falls, N.Y., 1988–90).

Antioxidant-Rich Foods

BETA-CAROTENE

Optimal amount: 10–30 mg per day. There is no established RDA.
Good sources: All colorful vegetables.
Supplements: 50–100 mg, if desired. Cigarette smokers should not take supplements.

	Serving Size	Beta-Carotene (mg)	% of Daily Recommendation (30 mg)
Vegetables			
brussels sprouts	1/2 cup	3.4	11
carrots	1 medium	12.2	41
collard greens	1/2 cup	1.0	3
kale	1/2 cup	8.2	27
mustard greens	1/2 cup	7.3	24
pumpkin	1/2 cup	16.1	54
spinach	1/2 cup	4.4	15
sweet potato	1 medium	2.9	10
turnips (cooked)	1/2 cup	2.4	8
Fruit			
apricots	3 medium	1.7	6
cantaloupe	1/2 medium	5.2	17
mango	1 medium	4.8	16
papaya	1 medium	3.7	12

BIOFLAVONOIDS

Optimal amount: Unknown.
Good sources: Fruit (especially apples), onions, tea (especially green tea), and red wine (a cup of tea or glass of red wine raises bioflavonoid levels in the blood for hours).

Antioxidant-Rich Foods, continued

VITAMIN C

Optimal amount: 100–400 mg per day. The RDA of 60 mg is well below the optimal intake.
Good sources: Many green vegetables and fruits.
Supplements: 100–400 mg, if desired.

	Serving Size	Vitamin C (mg)	% of Daily Requirement (60 mg)
Vegetables			
broccoli	1/2 cup	49	82
cabbage	1/2 cup	17	28
cauliflower	1/2 cup	34	57
chili pepper	1/2 cup	109	182
collard greens	1/2 cup	9	15
green pepper	1 medium	95	158
kale	1/2 cup	51	85
peas (canned)	1/2 cup	12	20
peas (fresh)	1/2 cup	38	63
potato (baked)	1 medium	26	43
sauerkraut	1/2 cup	17	28
winter squash	1/2 cup	10	17
Fruits			
cantaloupe	1/2 medium	113	188
grapefruit	1/2 medium	41	68
oranges	1 medium	70	117
papaya	1 medium	188	313
strawberries	1 cup	85	142

Antioxidant-Rich Foods, continued

VITAMIN E

Optimal amount: 30–100 mg per day. The RDA of 10 mg per day is well below the optimal intake.
Good sources: All whole grains and many vegetables and vegetable oils.
Supplements: 60–100 mg per day as a preventive measure; 300–800 mg per day for therapeutic purposes. Higher amounts should be monitored by a physician.

	Serving Size	Vitamin E (mg)	% of Daily Requirement (10 mg)
Grains and Grain Products			
brown rice	1/2 cup	1.2	12
seven-grain bread	1 slice	0.3	3
wheat bread	1 slice	0.2	2
white bread	1 slice	0.3	3
white rice	1/2 cup	0.4	4
wild rice	1/2 cup	1.8	18
Seeds and Nuts			
almonds	1 oz.	5.0	50
peanuts	1 oz.	3.1	31
sunflower seeds	1 oz.	14.8	148
Vegetables			
asparagus	1/2 cup	1.8	18
beets	1/2 cup	2.0	20
kidney beans	1/2 cup	4.4	44
pinto or lima beans (cooked)	1/2 cup	4.1	41
spinach (raw, frozen, or cooked)	1/2 cup	1.9	19
sweet potato*	1 medium	5.5	55
turnip	1/2 cup	1.8	18

Antioxidant-Rich Foods, continued

	Serving Size	Vitamin E (mg)	% of Daily Requirement (10 mg)
Fruits			
apple	1 medium	0.4	4
mango	1 medium	2.7	27
pear (canned)	1/2 medium	1.8	18
pear (fresh)	1 medium	1.3	13
Fish			
cod (canned, poached, or broiled)	3 oz.	0.8	8
mackerel	3 oz.	1.5	15
salmon (broiled or canned)	3 oz.	1.6–1.8	16–18
shrimp (broiled or fried)	3 oz.	0.6–3.5	6–35
Oils			
corn oil	1 tbsp.	11.2	112
margarine	1 tsp.	8.0	80
olive oil	1 tbsp.	1.9	19
safflower oil	1 tbsp.	5.5	55

*In contrast to sweet potatoes, yams have no vitamin E, and 1/2 cup of mashed potatoes has only 0.1 mg.

Antioxidant-Rich Foods, continued

VITAMIN B₆

Optimal amount: 1–2 mg per day.
Good sources: Whole grains, beans, nuts, fruit, meat.*
Supplements: 2 mg per day for pregnant women with more than one fetus or who are heavy smokers; 1 mg per day if needed for other adults.

	Serving Size	Vitamin B₆ (mg)	% of Daily Requirement (2 mg)
Vegetables			
garbanzo beans	1/2 cup	0.6	30
potato (baked)	1 medium	0.7	35
sweet potato	1 medium	0.3	15
Fruits			
avocado	1 medium	0.5–0.8	25–40
banana	1 medium	0.7	35
cantaloupe	1/2 medium	0.3	15
dates	10	0.2	10
figs (dried)	1 medium	0.4	20
raisins	1/2 cup	0.2	10
watermelon	1 cup	0.2	10
Grains			
brown rice	1/2 cup	0.1	5
rice bran	1/3 cup	1.1	55
white rice	1/2 cup	0.05	2–3
wild rice	1/2 cup	1.3	65
Meat			
liver	3 oz.	0.8	40

*Fava beans, broccoli, carrots, chili peppers, spinach, and okra each have 0.2 mg per serving, which comes out to 10% of RDA.

CHAPTER FIVE

Immune System
Booster #2: Minerals

M INERALS ARE THE tiny — in fact, imperceptible — rocks in your food. They are the same stuff that is gouged out of mines and used to construct buildings, make batteries, and conduct electricity. They are metals, composing much of the earth's crust. These bits of rock are unearthed by rain, rivers, and wind, carried to topsoils, and absorbed by plants, which are then eaten by animals and humans. Plants are the middlemen, so to speak, in the long journey these tiny metals make from the soil to your bloodstream and cells.

Minerals help build the proteins that combine to form the underlying structure for your bones, organs, muscles, and nerve tissue. Minerals are also needed to maintain the function of these tissues.

More than sixty minerals are used by the human body — together they compose about 4 percent of our total weight — but only twenty-two of them are considered essential. Seven of these — calcium, chlorine, magnesium, phosphorus, potassium, sodium, and sulfur — are present in our tissues in relatively large quantities and are therefore referred to as macrominerals. The other fifty or so are classified as trace minerals, meaning they are present in our tissues in relatively small amounts. Finally, the ultra trace minerals exist in our cells in only the tiniest quantities.

Such minute amounts might lead us to believe that they are relatively unimportant, but that would be incorrect. Like vitamins, minerals work synergistically with enzymes, other vitamins, and other minerals, making it possible for the body to utilize all essential nutrients and conduct normal cellular activity. For example, boron, a trace mineral found in fruits and vegetables (such as apples, pears, broccoli, and carrots) is found in the blood in only tiny amounts. Yet it is essential for the utilization and regulation of calcium, magnesium, and phosphorus — all macrominerals. Without boron, three of the major minerals that we hear so much about would not be much good to us.

Though minerals and vitamins are currently being studied assiduously, much about them is still unknown. However, what is known points directly to the need for a healthy and balanced diet, which is the only way to ensure that you will get all the nutrients you need, including those science still doesn't fully understand.

Minerals are essential to a vast array of metabolic and immune system functions and are therefore fundamental to human health. All of the minerals your body needs are available from vegetable sources alone, including whole grains, beans, leafy greens, roots, and fruit. In addition, fish, poultry, and red meat are abundant sources. However, red meat and certain parts of poultry are often rich in fat, which depresses the immune system. Therefore, we should mainly rely upon vegetable foods as a source of minerals, supplementing them occasionally with animal foods. The chart at the end of this chapter can help you make selections.

Though all the minerals used by the body are essential, only a handful have been proven to have clear immunity-related functions or specific roles in the protection against disease. These minerals are zinc, iron, copper, and magnesium. Here's what science has discovered about each of these minerals and their relationship to the immune system and individual illnesses.

Zinc and the Immune System

Zinc Deficiency

Zinc deficiency — the most common zinc-related problem in humans — is associated with a weakened immune response and greater susceptibility to infection. Unfortunately, the old and often false belief — if a little is good, a lot is better — is once again untrue. We need balanced zinc levels in our blood. Too much zinc is as depressing to the immune system as too little.

A zinc deficiency causes the thymus gland to atrophy, or shrink. The thymus is composed of compartments that produce T lymphocytes, including CD4 cells, the immune system's commanding general. These compartments shrink when zinc levels fall below normal, but after three to six months of supplementation, these compartments are restored to normal. In addition, zinc is used by the thymus to produce thymic hormones, which are needed to turn immature T lymphocytes into full-fledged, functional CD4 cells. When zinc levels are low, cysts sometimes form within the thymus. However, these cysts often disappear when zinc levels are normalized.

Outside the thymus gland, zinc deficiency has an independent effect on mature CD4 cells, causing fewer of them to appear in the blood. Inadequate zinc also makes existing CD4 cells less responsive to the presence of disease. They don't multiply as rapidly when confronted with an illness or infection, and they don't destroy diseases as aggressively as they do when zinc levels are optimal.

Nevertheless, the immune system bounces back when zinc

levels return to normal. CD4 cells respond to disease with their former ferocity, and the overall number of CD4 cells is returned to normal.

T cells are not the only immune cells that are impaired by inadequate zinc. Natural killer cells, so important in the fight against malignant cells and tumors, are significantly more sluggish in the face of cancer and other diseases. Illness thus has a greater chance of getting a foothold in the system.

When zinc is low, B cells don't produce adequate amounts of antibodies, which makes the immune response to a bacterium or virus less effective.

Causes of Zinc Deficiency

Zinc deficiency can occur in a number of ways, beginning with the failure of the small intestine to absorb enough of the mineral. Absorption can be hampered by excesses of other dietary components, notably the iron and phytates found in soy products, that interfere with zinc uptake. Theoretically, people who eat lots of soy products, such as vegetarians, should suffer from lower than normal zinc levels, but oddly this has not been demonstrated by researchers. In fact, a study of Seventh Day Adventists (who practice vegetarianism) showed that zinc intake and plasma levels were normal.

The people who most commonly have low zinc levels are intravenous drug abusers and alcoholics, especially alcoholics with cirrhosis of the liver. Other people at risk include patients with inflammatory bowel disease, adolescents, and the elderly. All three of these groups tend to follow narrow diets that may be inadequate in zinc. Convalescing adults experience higher than average demands for zinc because muscle tissue must be replaced. This, of course, places the elderly at even greater risk.

Low zinc also may occur because of excessive excretion of the mineral, which can be accelerated by estrogen, stress, and starvation. Women who use the pill and who frequently diet are at special risk. Certain drugs, such as isoniazid for TB and penicillamine, also can contribute to zinc deficiency.

How Zinc Affects Illness

Zinc and Infections

Children with inadequate zinc in their bloodstreams have been shown to have significantly higher rates of infection than those with adequate zinc. Also, studies have shown that colds don't last as long in people with adequate zinc, as compared to those with low zinc.

In animal studies, mice on low-zinc diets were less able to fight *Candida albicans* and parasitic infections, partly because of an impaired ability to produce cytokines and partly because of reduced killing by macrophages.

Zinc and Cancer

Although zinc's effect on cancer has been less well studied, it probably also plays a protective role for people with cancer. In animal studies, zinc supplementation slows the growth of tumor cells. Human studies indicate that zinc levels tend to be lower in patients with advanced cancers; these lower levels may contribute to the weakening of the immune system typically seen among patients with advanced cancers. The weakened immune response allows the cancer to grow more freely. It also makes cancer patients more susceptible to serious infections. At least one study showed that supplementation with zinc alone, or selenium and zinc together, improved T cell responses, granulocyte function, and levels of serum interferon in patients with advanced cancer.

Zinc and Other Illnesses

More generally, zinc deficiency is associated with weight loss, loss of the sense of taste and smell, amenorrhea (failure to menstruate), testicular retardation, rashes, and dwarfism.

Excess Zinc

Like other nutrients that are toxic at higher than normal levels, zinc too can impair the immune response when we take too much of it. Megadoses of zinc can also cause a secondary copper deficiency and adversely affect blood cholesterol levels. Additional hazards of excess zinc include nausea, vomiting, bleeding, and abdominal pain. In pregnant women it can cause premature labor and stillbirth.

Overconsumption of zinc, especially easy for those taking zinc supplements, is a lot more dangerous than most people think. It can mean the difference between being HIV-positive and progressing to full-blown AIDS. A recent study of HIV-positive men showed that even moderately high zinc intake was associated with an increased risk of HIV progression to AIDS.

The analysis divided the study participants into four groups based on different levels of zinc intake. Those who consumed the lowest levels of zinc, less than 11.6 milligrams per day, were the least likely to develop AIDS. However, the risk of developing AIDS increased as the zinc intake increased. This unexpected result is probably related to a paradoxical aspect of HIV infection: HIV replication requires higher levels of zinc. (We'll discuss this finding further in Chapter 15.)

Effects of Zinc When Combined with Other Minerals

As we said, minerals work together to create synergistic effects. Zinc and copper, for instance, are needed for the functioning of the enzyme superoxide dismutase, which destroys otherwise harmful oxidants.

Iron and the Immune System

Because immune cells have extensive mechanisms to control their iron reserves, they seem to function normally over a wide range of iron levels in the blood. Nevertheless, deficiencies and excesses do affect immune response.

Deficiencies of iron are associated with increased incidences of infections. The ability of macrophages to kill bacteria and viruses is reduced, and CD4 cells and natural killer cells are also weakened.

Nevertheless, the net effect of iron deficiency on the immune system for most adults appears small, and there is little evidence that infections and other diseases are increased when iron levels are low. The real problems occur when iron intake is excessive.

Excess Iron

Excess iron depresses the immune response. Although the effects on individual immune cells are not well understood, it is known that natural killer cell activity can be depressed, while suppressor T cells (CD8 cells) may increase in number. In short, the more suppressor cells there are, the more the immune system is held back or reined in by the CD8 cells. For these reasons, scientists generally recommend that adults not add iron supplements to their diets.

As immunologist John Kemp wrote in the *Journal of Clinical Immunology* (13:81–89, 1993), "Insofar as adults are concerned, however, the risks of [iron supplementation] probably outweigh the benefits. It thus appears that there is essentially no satisfactory rationale for routine iron supplementation unless significant iron deficiency has been specifically documented."

Copper and the Immune System

Copper is needed to form and maintain bones, blood vessels, and nerves and to sustain a healthy immune response. It also combines with iron to create red blood cells. Copper deficiencies are uncommon because the mineral is so widely available in foods; most unprocessed food contains copper in adequate quantities to ensure health.

Severe copper deficiencies have been shown to affect immune function, but most of the data demonstrating such effects are from animal studies. It is not known if small or marginal copper deficiency affects immunity.

Magnesium and the Immune System

Magnesium is involved in so many metabolic processes that it is essential for the health of every cell in the body. Fortunately, it is also abundant in a wide assortment of vegetable and animal foods, so deficiencies are uncommon and, when they do appear, are easily corrected.

Magnesium plays an interesting role in the immune response. In effect, it acts as a sort of human Velcro, an ability that is known as an adhesion reaction. Immune cells get around in the body by traveling through the bloodstream. In order for immune cells to be attracted to the areas at which they are needed, they develop adhesion molecules, substances that allow them to stick to places within the body so that they remain in place to deal with a particular problem.

For example, suppose you bruised your knee and have developed a minor infection. The cells within your knee's blood vessels will develop new proteins on their surfaces that make these cells sticky. These proteins are referred to as adhesion molecules, or integrins. When immune cells become activated, they also make their own integrins. Now you've got Velcro at the site of the bruise and on the immune cells that are traveling nearby. As the immune cells circulate through the body, they adhere to the sticky patches on the blood vessels near sites of inflammation. Now they can begin the work of destroying the intruding organisms. The adhesion molecules are also needed to help immune cells stick to cells carrying viruses or bacteria. Once they stick to their target, the immune cells can kill the invader.

Magnesium is essential to the work of integrins. Nevertheless, despite the importance of this mineral, there is no evidence as yet for a clinical effect of magnesium deficiency in humans. However, an upset in the ratio of calcium to magnesium can impair the nervous system.

Selenium and the Immune System

Selenium, a trace element, acts as an antioxidant. It also combines with other nutrients to activate glutathione's antioxidant properties. Small increases in selenium have been shown to boost production of CD4 cells and natural killer cells. Selenium also increases production of interferon and stimulates B cells to produce more antibodies.

Selenium and Cancer

Selenium's role as an antioxidant may be why it is associated with lower rates of cancer among those who eat adequate quantities of the mineral. Animal studies have shown that selenium intake is associated with a lower incidence of breast tumors. Several years ago, selenium was celebrated as a nutrient with profound cancer-protective properties. However, new research has suggested that although selenium is indeed a cancer inhibitor, it may not have the independent protective effects that scientists once believed. As in its relationship with glutathione, selenium's main role may be to combine with other nutrients, which work together to protect against cancer. In any case, much remains to be learned about selenium's role in cancer prevention. Until that time, it is better to derive this nutrient from its many food sources, rather than taking it as a supplement.

Selenium and Mental Function

Adequate selenium intake may be associated with emotional health and well-being. Researchers David Benton and Richard Cook, at University College in Swansea, Wales, have found that people who eat the least amount of selenium suffer higher rates of anxiety, depression, and fatigue. When these same people increased their selenium intake, their moods and energy levels improved.

Excess selenium can be toxic, which makes supplementation of selenium unwise.

■ ■ ■

Minerals are vitally important to the immune system and to overall health. Much remains mysterious about these tiny, yet powerful particles. Until we learn more, however, it benefits us all to eat a mineral-rich diet, which, fortunately, is easy to create.

Mineral-Rich Foods

ZINC

Optimal amount: 15–20 mg per day for men; 12–18 mg per day for women.
Good sources: Grains, shellfish, meat, and beans.

	Serving Size	Zinc (mg)	% of Daily Requirement (12 mg)
Grains			
fortified cereals*	1 oz.	15.0	125
granola	1 oz.	1.0	8
millet	1 cup	2.9	24

Mineral-Rich Foods, continued

	Serving Size	Zinc (mg)	% of Daily Requirement (12 mg)
Shellfish			
crab (steamed)	3 oz.	7.0	58
eastern oysters	6 medium	76.0	633
shrimp	3 oz.	1.3	11
Meat			
chicken breast	3 oz.	1.0	8
ground beef	3 oz.	6.0	50
rib-eye steak	3 oz.	6.0	50
roast beef	3 oz.	6.0	50
turkey (dark meat without skin)	3 oz.	3.8	32
Beans			
baked beans	1/2 cup	1.8	15
pinto beans	1/2 cup	1.2	10

*Not all cold cereals are good sources of zinc. Corn flakes, for example, contain none. Consult the nutritional information on the cereal box.

IRON

Optimal amount: 15 mg per day for women who menstruate; 10 mg per day for men and all other women.
Good sources: Certain meats and fish, and certain vegetables, seaweeds, beans, and grains.
Supplements: Not recommended.

	Serving Size	Iron (mg)	% of Daily Requirement (15 mg)
Meat and Fish			
liver	3 oz.	7.5	50
rib-eye steak	3 oz.	2.2	15

Mineral-Rich Foods, continued

	Serving Size	Iron (mg)	% of Daily Requirement (15 mg)
sardines	3 oz. (about 15)	2.5	17
shrimp	3 oz.	2.6	17
Vegetables, Beans, and Grains			
millet	1 cup	5.7	38
peas	1/2 cup	1.9	13
pinto beans	1/2 cup	2.7	18
potato with skin	1 medium	2.7	18
spinach	1/2 cup	3.2	21
tofu (soybean curd)	1/2 cup	6.6	44

COPPER

Optimal amount: 1.5–3 mg per day.
Good sources: Red meat, shellfish, nuts, fruit, beans, raisins, and mushrooms.

MAGNESIUM

Optimal amount: 350 mg per day for men; 280 mg per day for women.
Good sources: Whole grains, leafy green vegetables, beans, nuts, and fruit.

	Serving Size	Magnesium (mg)	% of Daily Requirement (350 mg)
Vegetables and Beans			
fava beans	1/2 cup	88	25
potato (baked)	1 medium	55	16
spinach	1/2 cup	79	23
tofu	1/2 cup	127	36
Fish			
cod	3 oz.	36	10
escargot	3 oz.	147	42

Mineral-Rich Foods, continued

	Serving Size	Magnesium (mg)	% of Daily Requirement (350 mg)
halibut	3 oz.	91	26
oysters	6 medium	37	11
Nuts and Grains			
almonds	1 oz.	85	24
bran flakes	1 oz.	60	17
millet	1 cup	137	39
peanuts	1 oz.	53	15

SELENIUM

Optimal amount: 70 mg per day for men; 55 mg per day for women.
Good sources: Wheat, other whole grains, nuts and seeds, and fish.
Supplements: Not recommended.

CHAPTER SIX

Immune System Booster #3: A Low-Fat Diet

F AT IS A DIRTY WORD in the nutritional lexicon. It contributes to or causes the most widespread and deadly diseases in the Western world. The typical American diet, which is based primarily on animal foods such as red meat, dairy products, and eggs, virtually guarantees that people will eat enough fat to depress their immune systems and eventually bring on a serious illness, such as heart disease, cancer, adult-onset diabetes, obesity, cataracts, Parkinson's disease, and Alzheimer's disease.

In an effort to reduce fat, Americans have cut down on their consumption of red meat, but many unwittingly have turned to other high-fat foods, including cheese, whole milk, and high-fat desserts. Hence, fat intake, although dropping slowly, remains high and consequently causes millions to suffer from preventable diseases and being overweight.

In China, the average fat consumption is approximately 14.5 percent of the total diet — less than half of what most Americans consume. For those who follow a low-fat diet, the incidence of heart disease, cancer, and other degenerative diseases is remarkably low. However, those Chinese who eat high-fat diets — some Chinese eat far more meat than the average citizen does — experience the same diseases we in the West experience. In fact, this same trend exists in the United States. Those who eat diets low in fat — 30 percent or less — have lower rates of disease.

Fortunately, fat consumption is very much in our control and therefore can be both a powerful and important tool for boosting the immune system.

Fat, Energy, Calories, and Longevity

An adult primarily needs energy from his or her diet, and the best source of energy is carbohydrates, especially complex carbohydrates, which come from unrefined grains, vegetables, and fruit. Simple carbohydrates, also known as simple sugars, burn rapidly, and quickly leave an adult in an energy-depleted state. Complex carbohydrates burn slowly and provide long-lasting energy. Therefore, carbohydrates — and not fat-rich foods — should be the mainstay of our diets.

There are three types of fat: *saturated* fat, found in all animal products and a few vegetables; *polyunsaturated* fats, found in grains, seeds, vegetables, fruit, and fish (fish also have saturated fats, but much less than other animal foods); and *monounsaturated* fats, found in olives and nuts. Chemically, these fats differ in the amount of hydrogen atoms found in the fat molecule. That molecule consists of oxygen, carbon, and hydrogen. The more hydrogen that is present in the fat molecule, the more saturated it is. Saturated fats tend to be solid at room temperature. Polyunsaturated and monounsaturated fats are liquid at room temperature.

Saturated fats cause blood cholesterol levels to rise, triggering the onset of cholesterol plaques within arteries, also known as atherosclerosis. They have also been shown to cause cancer and other life-threatening illnesses. Polyunsaturated fats tend to lower blood cholesterol — including LDL cholesterol — and also prevent blood from clotting. Monounsaturated fats tend to have a small cholesterol-lowering effect. Excessive amounts of polyunsaturated fats also depress the immune system and have been linked to cancer.

The primary role of fat is to serve as a secondary source of energy, to be used when carbohydrate stores are depleted. Your body will first burn all the carbohydrates — in whatever form you eat them — and store the fat you eat in your adipose tissues, located below the surface of your skin. Consequently, all fats add both calories and weight to the body. Fat, in effect, is your energy savings account. It's not your primary fuel.

Fat is essential for metabolizing vitamins A, D, E, and K (the so-called fat-soluble vitamins) and creating hormones, including prostaglandins, which help to control blood pressure and inflammation. Prostaglandins also play a role in regulating the immune response. Finally, fats (also known as *lipids*), are an integral part of the cell membrane. They maintain fluidity of the membrane and must be kept in balance within the cell's outer structure so that communication between the cell's receptors and its nucleus can be maintained. All of these functions require very little fat.

Fat is the most calorically dense nutrient in our diets. A gram of carbohydrate contains four calories; a gram of fat contains nine calories. Research has shown that people who consume diets low in calories live longer than those on high-calorie diets. Since fat is loaded with calories, it follows that those who eat low-fat diets tend to eat fewer calories and thus enhance their chances at longevity.

All fats depress the immune system when consumed in excess. Polyunsaturated and monounsaturated fats can be just as bad as saturated fats if we eat too much of them. The great majority of vegetable sources, however, is significantly lower in fat than animal foods, and therefore can generally be consumed in greater quantity without adding much fat to the diet.

Fat and Your Immune System

Excessive consumption of fat hits the immune system with a devastating one-two punch: on the one hand, fat is a free radical producer, causing cell mutations and atherosclerosis; on the other, it depresses the immune system, which weakens your body's efforts to fight the disease-causing effects of fat.

Every immune cell is surrounded by a membrane equipped with antenna-like receptors that capture information from outside the cell to determine the presence of nearby threats to the body. Once a threat is recognized, the cell passes the information through the cell's membrane and on to the nucleus, which then instructs the cell on how to respond to the threat.

The cell membrane is composed of approximately 50 percent protein and 50 percent lipids. That delicate balance between protein and fat is altered when you eat excessive amounts of fat. As it becomes clogged with fat, the cell membrane becomes less fluid and therefore less conductive of sensory information, which means that the immune cell cannot pass information from its receptors to the cell's nucleus, or brain center. Without such information, cells don't know how to respond to invading bacteria, viruses, or cancer cells. The effects of this breakdown in communication are varied and widespread.

CD4 Cells and Fat

You might say that fat puts the immune system to sleep, or at least makes it lazy. Studies have shown that fat prevents CD4 cells from multiplying as rapidly in the presence of disease. Perhaps worse, moderate- to high-fat diets (high fat being about 41 percent of calories) *reduce by half* the ability of CD4 cells and natural killer cells to kill cancer cells and tumors!

Macrophages and Fat

Macrophages recognize antigens and cancer cells by touching them with their receptors and sensitive cell membranes. Unfortunately, fat infiltrates the cell membranes of macrophages and reduces their sensitivity to threatening substances and cells. This, of course, allows the threatening agents to proliferate and grow stronger before the immune system mounts an attack.

Fish Oils and Immunity

Fish oils contain omega-3 polyunsaturated fat, which reduces blood cholesterol levels. They also make the blood less sticky, which prevents the formation of blood clots inside the arteries. These clots, known as thrombi (plural of thrombus), cause most heart attacks and strokes. These benefits have made fish oil seem like a kind of panacea for heart disease. However, large amounts of fish oil are needed to lower cholesterol (sometimes as much as seventy-five to one hundred grams taken daily, or nearly four ounces), and that fish oil can depress the immune system.

Fish oils inhibit the production of chemical messengers inside your immune system (specifically interleukin-1 and tumor necrosis factor). This made some scientists think that fish oils would be beneficial in the treatment of arthritis, a disorder characterized by inflammation. In fact, subsequent studies did find that fish oils reduced the swelling and joint pain of people with arthritis.

However, the decrease in chemical messengers definitely has a dark side. How many of us want to have reduced levels of interleukin-1 and tumor necrosis factor, both of which are essential in the fight against viruses and cancer? And these were not the only areas of concern. A study published in *The Journal of Leukocyte Biology* (December 1993) showed that the same daily intake of fish oils (eighteen grams) suppressed lymphocyte multiplication by as much as 70 percent.

All the benefits of fish oil can be accomplished by sharply reducing intake of fat and cholesterol. A low-fat diet protects against heart disease and cancer while it boosts immunity. It makes the blood less sticky and thus less likely to form blood clots and thrombi. And finally, research suggests that such a diet may even offer protection against autoimmune disorders, such as arthritis.

Low-Fat Diet and Arthritis

Scientists have long suspected that diet plays a crucial role in the onset of arthritis, but the elimination of individual foods has never presented convincing results. Scientists in Norway took a different approach. In a study published in *The Lancet* (October 12, 1991), scientists compared the effects of two different diets on two groups of people with rheumatoid arthritis. The first group, composed of twenty-seven people, followed a strict vegetarian regimen, whereas the control group, consisting of twenty-six people, followed a standard high-fat diet.

Those on the vegetarian diet proceeded through a three-stage regimen. The first stage, which lasted for seven days, included only vegetable foods, but mostly in the form of vegetable broths. The subjects also consumed vegetable juices, herbal teas, and garlic. During the second stage, which lasted for three and a half months, the group ate only vegetables and avoided all red meat, eggs, dairy foods, citrus fruits, refined sugars, spices, salt, and grains containing gluten (such as wheat). After they followed this regimen for four months, dairy foods were gradually reintroduced into the diet. A new dairy food was added every other day, until the final diet consisted of vegetable foods, certain whole grains, and dairy products. That diet was followed for one year. Both the subjects on the vegetarian diet and the controls kept diaries of what they ate, also noting any changes in their symptoms.

The results were nothing short of remarkable. After one month, the people following the vegetarian diet reported significant decreases in the number of swollen and tender joints.

They also experienced significantly less joint stiffness, especially in the morning, and fewer flare-ups of symptoms. The vegetarians also reported feeling stronger and healthier overall. Remarkably, these improvements lasted throughout the entire thirteen-month study.

By comparison, the control group suffered their usual arthritis symptoms — the pain and swelling had even grown worse for many. The researchers concluded that a period of fasting, followed by a vegetarian diet, substantially decreased the symptoms of arthritis.

Calories and Immune Response

As we mentioned earlier, calorie consumption seems to have an independent effect on the immune system. The average male in the United States eats approximately twenty-five hundred calories per day, and the average female about eighteen hundred calories per day. Many people, of course, eat much more than the average, shown by the fact that fully one quarter of Americans are obese. In fact, the body needs far fewer calories to maintain normal metabolism and health. Animal studies have shown that when calories are restricted to half the normal amount, longevity is increased significantly, even among animals that have autoimmune disorders and short life spans. Life spans increase for animals even when the calorie-restricted diet is composed of 80 percent protein. Calorie restriction greatly reduces the percentage of animals that develop leukemia after radiation, as well. In one study, less than one tenth of the animals on restricted diets developed leukemia, compared to those eating high-calorie diets.

Fat, which is a major source of calories, seems to have an independent effect as well. Studies have shown that when calories and fat are analyzed separately for their effect on longevity, fat intake has the greater impact on health and death rates. Fat seems to weaken the system in a number of ways, and one of them is to add unhealthy quantities of calories.

At the University of Texas Health Science Center in San Antonio, Dr. Gabriel Fernandes, an immunologist, has shown that lowering fat consumption in animals significantly reduced the risk of their developing immunological deficiency diseases and cancer. He also showed that when placed on a low-fat diet, mice experienced a reduction in age-related diseases and immune system depression — even in a strain of mice genetically predisposed to immune system deficiency and cancer.

Dr. Robert Good, an immunologist at the Oklahoma Medical Research Foundation in Oklahoma City, has said that there is "now abundant evidence that even genetically determined diseases may be modified or even entirely prevented by limiting protein, calories, or fat content of the diet."

Fat and Cancer

Research has linked both total fat intake, as well as the type of fat eaten, to the incidence of cancer, especially cancers of the breast, colon, ovaries, and prostate. Much of the evidence comes from cross-cultural, or epidemiological, studies. In nations where fat consumption is low, cancer rates are low; but in countries where fat intake is high, cancer rates are also high. Research has shown that when people who eat low-fat diets in their native countries, such as the Japanese, immigrate to the United States and adopt a more Western, high-fat diet, their cancer rates increase to equal those of Americans.

The source of fat also appears to be important. Animal fats (fish oil less so than others) are associated with higher rates of cancer than vegetable fats. Studies suggest that fish oils and olive oil may actually reduce the incidence of cancer.

This research is suggestive rather than definitive, however. It's hard to draw direct conclusions from epidemiological research because many subtle differences in diet and lifestyle cannot easily be compared between countries.

When one looks at studies within one country, the association of fats and cancer, particularly breast cancer, is less clear. For instance, studies within Western nations have not shown a convincing association between higher breast cancer rates and total fat intake. When women with breast cancer were compared to women without breast cancer, it was found that total fat intake did not seem to differ between the two groups. However, certain correlations did seem important, such as the levels of saturated fat these women consumed. One study showed that for every 5 percent increase in saturated fat consumption, there was a 50 percent increased risk of dying of breast cancer.

Nevertheless, other factors support the link between fat intake and cancer, particularly breast cancer. Fat cells produce estrogen, and studies have shown that women with breast cancer have higher estrogen levels than women who are free of the disease. The more fat women eat, the more estrogen their bodies produce. Thus, women on high-fat diets have higher than average estrogen levels, placing them at greater risk.

Lowering Estrogen Naturally

One of the ways estrogen levels can be lowered is by increasing one's intake of fiber, which binds with estrogen and eliminates it through the bowel. By eating a diet that is low in fat and high in fiber, a woman can substantially reduce her risk of contracting breast cancer.

Research has shown that many malignant breast tumors are dependent upon estrogen; when estrogen levels are significantly reduced, the tumors regress. This is the basis for the use of the drug tamoxifen as a treatment for breast cancer; tamoxifen reduces the effect of estrogens on cells. However, one of the best and fastest ways to lower estrogens in the blood is to change your diet, specifically by lowering fat and increasing fiber. The effects of such changes are dramatic.

In one study, women with high estrogen levels were placed on a high-fiber, low-fat diet and saw their estrogen levels drop by 50 percent in twenty-two days on the diet. That represents a remarkable drop in both estrogen and the risk of breast cancer.

Much more research needs to be done to clarify the effects of fat and fiber on breast cancer. Nevertheless, until all the data are gathered and analyzed, the best advice is to be prudent with fat consumption, especially saturated fat from animal sources. Women should keep their fat intake below 25 percent of total calories. Moreover, women with breast cancer should reduce their fat consumption to below 20 percent.

Fat and Heart Disease

Most of us do not think of heart disease as related to the immune system, but indeed it is. Fat is converted by the liver into low-density lipoproteins, or LDL cholesterol. Once in the bloodstream, these LDL particles oxidize and become free radicals. Macrophage cells recognize the decaying LDL particles as a waste product and begin to phagocytize, or gobble them up. The macrophages then become bloated with LDL and sink to the walls of the arteries, where they become embedded. Meanwhile, the ingested LDL particles, which decay inside the macrophage, deform both the macrophage cells and the artery wall. There, they form the first layer of scar tissue, known as a fatty streak, which is the first stage of atherosclerosis. As more fat and cholesterol are consumed, more macrophage cells consume the LDL particles, become bloated with decaying free radicals, and form even larger growths inside the artery. These growths eventually become volatile boils, or plaques, which can become so large that they block the artery passageway, thus preventing blood and oxygen from flowing to the heart or brain. This chain of events can lead to a heart attack or a stroke.

■ ■ ■

The link between high fat and heart disease is well established. It is becoming more clear, however, that different types of fats have very different effects on blood cholesterol levels. All forms of saturated fats, including partially hydrogenated fats in shortenings and margarine, clearly raise blood cholesterol levels and form the basis for atherosclerosis. The National Cholesterol Education Panel (NCEP) recommends that saturated fats be reduced from the current average of 14 percent of total caloric intake to approximately 4 percent. Polyunsaturated fats reduce cholesterol and make the blood less sticky, and thus less likely to form cholesterol plaques. The NCEP recommends that Americans replace most of their saturated fats with polyunsaturated fats, which would mean raising the current level of vegetable oils from the average of 6 percent of caloric intake to 10 percent. Finally, monounsaturated fats, which appear to have a neutral effect on blood cholesterol, should be decreased from the current average of 14 percent to 10 percent. Overall this would mean a suggested reduction from about 36 percent to 25 percent in fat consumption.

Certain vegetable oils, such as corn oil and safflower oil, have the added benefit of being very rich sources of vitamin E. Also, olive oil — a monounsaturated fat — is gaining scientific support as having health-protective qualities, particularly as it is used in Mediterranean diets. A 1994 study (twenty-seven months in length) found that women who consumed more olive oil had fewer deaths by heart attack and fewer nonfatal heart attacks.

They also had higher levels of vitamins A and E in their blood. Although this result is intriguing, it is too early to say if it was indeed the olive oil that was responsible for fewer heart attacks or if it was another associated factor.

■ ■ ■

All of us should be careful about our intake of fat — no matter what its source. We recommend that people get their fats primarily from vegetable sources and that they limit consumption of all oils. However, when faced with a choice between a saturated fat and a poly- or monounsaturated fat, choose the vegetable fat over the saturated fat every time.

By limiting fat, we'll make a quantum leap in our race against all serious diseases, in part because it will give our immune systems a big boost.

Calculating Fat in the Diet

A person eating two thousand calories per day should obtain four hundred to five hundred calories from fat. To translate this number into grams of fat, divide by nine, since there are approximately nine calories per gram of fat. The answer is approximately forty-four to fifty-five grams of fat per day.

Use the following table as a guide, and take the time to look at the nutritional information on food packages to help you make low-fat choices. Lowering fats reduces the risks of cancer and heart disease, and can help improve autoimmune diseases, particularly rheumatoid arthritis.

Sources of Fat

RED MEAT, CHICKEN, AND FISH[1]		
	Serving Size	Grams of Fat
chicken breast (without skin)	3 oz.	3.1
ground beef	3 oz.[2]	17.8
ground beef (lean)	3 oz.	14.0
mackerel	3 oz.	15.0
rib-eye steak	3 oz.	9.9
salmon	3 oz.	6.4
scrod	3 oz.	0.7
shrimp	3 oz.	1.7
sirloin steak	3 oz.	8.0
DAIRY PRODUCTS[3]		
American cheese	1 oz.	8.8
blue cheese	1 oz.	8.1
brie	1 oz.	7.8
butter	1 tsp.	4.1
cheddar cheese	1 oz.	9.3
ice cream	1/2 cup	5.0–18.0
margarine	1 tsp.	11.4
milk (whole)	8 oz.	8.2
milk with 1% fat	8 oz.	2.6
milkshake	16 fl. oz.	9.5
mozzarella	1 oz.	6.1
yogurt (low-fat plain)	1 cup	3.5
yogurt with fruit	1 cup	5.5
CRACKERS AND SNACKS*		
corn chips	1 oz.	10.0
microwave popcorn	3 cups	5.0[4]
potato chips	1 oz.	10.0

Sources of Fat, continued

	Serving Size	Grams of Fat
rice cakes	1	0
Ritz crackers	3	2.9
rye crisps	1	0
saltines	4	1.4
wheat thins	8	3.0
SWEETS*		
apple pie	1/8 of 9″ pie	13.0
apple turnover	1	19.3
chocolate chip cookies	1 (2″ diameter)	2.1
fig bars	2	1.0
fruit danish	1	13.0
fruit muffin	1 small	5.0
gingersnaps	2	1.1
granola	1 oz.	5.6
jelly donut	1	18.4
molasses cookies	2	2.9
pecan pie	1/8 of 9″ pie	29.3
vanilla wafers	2	7.0
NUTS[5]		
almonds	1 oz.	14.5
chestnuts	1 oz.	0.2
macadamias	1 oz.	20.6
peanuts	1 oz.	13.8
pecans	1 oz.	18.0

1. All except shrimp and scrod contain saturated fats.
2. A 3-oz. serving is typical for a sandwich. Dinner-size portions of these meats would likely weigh in at 6 oz.
3. Most contain saturated fats.
4. 0.3 g if air-popped.
5. Nuts tend to be high in monounsaturated fats.
* Type of fat used varies. Check packaging.

CHAPTER SEVEN

Immune System Booster #4: Medicinal Herbs, Spices, and Cancer-Fighting Foods

I F THERE IS ANYTHING in medicine that completes the circle between the ancient and the modern, it is the use of medicinal plants. The oral and written tradition that forms the foundation of herbology is, of course, many thousands of years old. Such knowledge has been used successfully to treat more people around the world than any other form of medicine. Today, our study of herbs and other specific health-promoting foods is essentially a reexamination — albeit from a scientific perspective — of our own inheritance from the great healers of old: Hippocrates, Galen, Avicenna, Paracelsus, and the mythical Yellow Emperor of China. The scientific search for knowledge is very much in partnership with traditional healers, for they are the ones who have singled out specific plants as having healing properties. These plants have gained special attention in the laboratory.

We in the West are committed to using science to determine the efficacy of a given therapy, and thus we are committed to relearning the use of medicinal plants from our own perspective. Many books describe the use of medicinal plants from a traditional perspective; we are reporting the scientific documentation, where it exists, of the efficacy of these therapies and fostering the safest possible use of medicinal plants.

A note of caution is in order when using medicinal plants. They sometimes contain potent chemicals that can have profound effects on the body. In proper doses they can relieve symptoms and cause stimulation, relaxation, or cleansing, but in excess they can lead to vomiting, headaches, diarrhea, convulsions, liver damage, and coma. Also, since their production is not regulated, some preparations may become contaminated with lead, thallium, aconite, or other dangerous substances. Such contaminants have been associated with problems ranging from hair loss to liver and heart damage, and they can lead to death. We have chosen to discuss the safest herbs available and the most widely studied.

Another warning: certain spices that have been demonstrated as being supportive to the immune system can also cause allergies in certain people. These flavorings include curry and ginger. Beyond the points that we report in this chapter and in Part III, no harmful side effects result from any of the medicinal plants that we discuss as far as we know.

Another concern related to using herbs is that the strength of a plant's active ingredients depends on the conditions under which the plant is grown, which makes the effective dose subject to guesswork or trial and error. We strongly recommend that you obtain herbs only from reputable sources and that you mention their use to your health care provider, particularly if new symptoms develop. For instance, some plants cause symptoms similar to those associated with AIDS-related complex (ARC) in HIV-infected people, which could be misleading to both patient and physician.

With that in mind, let's examine the evidence. As you will see, researchers are discovering that a scientific basis exists for much traditional practice and folklore concerning medicinal plants.

Shiitake Mushrooms

The shiitake mushroom (of the genus *Lentinula*) is a wide, flat-capped mushroom traditionally grown in Asia and now widely available throughout the United States and Europe. For centuries, it has been used in Asian cuisine as a delicious and health-enhancing food. In the past two decades, the shiitake mushroom has grown in popularity throughout the West, thanks to the upscale restaurants that offer the succulent-tasting mushroom as an exotic side dish and to people familiar with its traditional medicinal uses. Today, science is documenting its varied and powerful effects on the immune system and its ability to protect against heart disease and cancer.

Shiitake mushrooms are high in protein (13–18 percent) and contain niacin, thiamine, riboflavin, and a polysaccharide called *lentinan* that has been approved in Japan as an anticancer drug. Recent research has shown that lentinan stimulates macrophages and natural killer cells to destroy cancer cells and tumors.

Another substance isolated in shiitake mushrooms, called cortinelin, has proved to be an effective broad-spectrum antibiotic. Also, compounds known as sulfides in shiitake mushrooms can kill ringworm, fungus, and other causes of skin disease.

Studies at the U.S. National Cancer Institute and the Japanese National Cancer Institute have established the shiitake mushroom as a cancer fighter, a booster of the immune system, and a powerful cholesterol-lowering food. It also inhibits virus replication. Scientists at Japan's Yamaguchi University School of Medicine have found that shiitake mushroom extract protected cells against the destruction normally caused by HIV infection. The scientists went on to recommend that shiitake mushrooms be used in conjunction with other AIDS treatments.

Goro Chihara, a leading Japanese researcher on lentinan, says that the substance "prolongs the life span of patients with advanced and recurrent stomach, colorectal, and breast cancer."

Shiitake Mushrooms and Heart Disease

The pioneer of shiitake research, Kisaku Mori, Ph.D., founded the Institute of Mushroom Research in Tokyo. Mori documented the healing effects of the shiitake mushroom and tried to isolate its most active compounds.

One of those compounds, called eritadenine, has been shown by both American and Japanese researchers to dramatically lower blood cholesterol. Studies have shown that eating three ounces (five or six mushrooms) per day can lower blood cholesterol by 12 percent in one week. Other research has suggested that the cholesterol-lowering effect of shiitake mushroom extract — the concentrated form of the mushroom — may be as much as 25 percent when used over a couple of weeks.

Shiitake mushrooms are widely available in supermarkets and natural foods stores. They can be used in soups, stews, and vegetable medleys — steamed, boiled, or sautéed. We recommend eating two to six mushrooms per week (or two to four, if you are also using reishi mushrooms).

Reishi Mushrooms

A medicinal mushroom used traditionally in China is reishi *(Ganoderma lucidium),* most widely used to enhance the function of the immune system. It has been shown to cause lymphocytes to multiply rapidly in the face of a disease-causing agent, as well as trigger production of interleukin-2. Reishi also promotes the creation of adhesion molecules that help to gather immune cells in a specific location where they are needed. Reishi also stimulates the production of tumor necrosis factor. Its extract is widely available in natural foods and health food stores; the mushroom itself is common in Asian food markets and some natural foods stores. We recommend eating two to four mushrooms per week.

Garlic

Garlic has been celebrated for centuries in both the East and the West as a powerful health enhancer. Today, modern science is discovering the biochemical reasons for this strong-smelling herb's reputation, especially as an anti-infection and anticancer agent.

Garlic contains thiol compounds that stimulate the body's detoxifying activities. These compounds include allicin (the most widely known), ajoene, s-allylmercaptocysteine, and allyl alcohol. Allicin is most effective when eaten raw, but researchers at the National Cancer Institute say that garlic has health-promoting effects even after it is cooked.

Many of these same chemicals are also found in onions, though apparently in smaller quantities. "It seems that the stronger the food — and in the case of garlic, that means the smell — the stronger the health-enhancing effects are," says Michael Wargovich, M.D., a professor of medicine at M. D. Anderson Cancer Center in Houston and an expert on garlic.

Garlic and the Immune System

Garlic extracts boost a number of immune activities that could be related to controlling cancer. They stimulate T cell proliferation and enhance natural killer cell activity. It promotes both the proliferation and the efficiency of interleukin-2. In another set of experiments, garlic extracts were shown to strengthen the oxidative bursts of macrophages. Macrophages use these bursts of oxidants to kill bacteria, cancer cells, and virus-producing cells. Garlic has also been demonstrated as an effective antibacterial and antiviral agent.

Garlic and Cancer

Garlic may have anticancer effects that are independent of the immune system, though the exact mechanisms by which garlic may protect against cancer, and even attack cancer cells and tumors, have yet to be fully understood.

Epidemiological research shows an association of high garlic consumption and lower rates of gastric cancer (cancers of the stomach, intestinal tract, and rectum) in Italian and Chinese populations.

Garlic has been shown to protect lipids (fats and cholesterol in the blood) from being oxidized, thus preventing the onset of free radical formation, the cause of most degenerative diseases. In fact, garlic extracts have been shown to decrease the development of cancer even after exposure to powerful carcinogens such as radiation.

Garlic is thought to have a role in detoxifying carcinogens. According to Dr. Wargovich, garlic enhances the liver's ability to metabolize and neutralize carcinogens that would otherwise produce cancer cells and tumors. Garlic stimulates the liver to more effectively identify these poisons and turn them into harmless, water-soluble compounds.

Garlic also encourages a variety of detoxifying enzymes to be produced by the body, some of which directly attack cancer cells and tumors. Scientists speculate that garlic may block the effects of a certain group of fatty acids called prostaglandins, which are hormone-like substances. Prostaglandins may encourage tumor growth when they are unchecked.

As if this was not enough, garlic compounds also inhibit the formation of thrombi by inhibiting platelet aggregation. They apparently block adhesion through integrins on the platelet surface. This might reduce the risk of strokes and cardiovascular disease.

Finally, garlic is also a good source of selenium.

Use garlic three or more times per week, raw or cooked, and preferably in both forms. Cooked garlic works well in pasta and vegetable dishes and as a condiment on bread; raw, it can be served with vegetables and salads.

Licorice

A less touted herbal food — though one the child in all of us will be happy to rediscover — is licorice. A polysaccharide, licorice extract called glycyrrhizin is used clinically and is said to have anti-inflammatory, antitumor, and antiviral effects. In addition to glycyrrhizin, licorice root can contain ten different bioflavonoids, compounds that boost the immune system and fight cancer.

Licorice should be avoided by people with heart problems, hypertension, obesity, or kidney problems. The herb serves as a stimulant to the heart and circulation, which can be taxing on people with cardiovascular disease.

Licorice intake should be limited to two to three ounces of licorice candy per day to avoid problems with swelling, increased blood pressure, and vomiting. We recommend one cup of licorice tea per day, three or more times per week, when you are affected by a cold or flu. At other times, use it occasionally as an immune system booster and another way of protecting yourself against cancer. Licorice tea bags are widely available in natural foods and health food stores.

Echinacea

Echinacea *(Echinacea compositae)* is among the most commonly used medicinal herbs in the world today. Long known for its ability to boost the immune system, which is now being backed up by scientific research, echinacea has been consistently shown to increase the ability of macrophages and granulocytes to phagocytize bacteria or virus-producing cells. Studies have demonstrated that these effects could be increased by giving echinacea in combination with extracts from other herbs, including *Eupatorium perfoliatum, Baptisia tinctoria,* and *Arnica montana.*

Animal studies have shown that echinacea increases production of interleukin-1, interleukin-6, and tumor necrosis factor by macrophages, all of which offer increased protection against infections by several parasitic organisms, including the yeast *Candida albicans.* Echinacea also has anti-inflammatory properties and stimulates CD4 cells to multiply more vigorously in the face of a disease-causing agent.

Echinacea may work best when taken in small doses over a short period of time, such as once or twice a day for one to three days. At that point, it may be preferable to allow the herb to do its work without giving any more doses. In one study, one moderate dose was followed by a week without echinacea. This single dose stimulated lymphocyte proliferation and caused a reaction to a standard skin test, which showed that the immune system was boosted and highly reactive when challenged. However, higher doses of the herb, given over several days, seemed to suppress both the proliferation of T cells and a reaction to skin testing. Traditional herbalists often recommend that echinacea be used twice a day, for one to three days, and then stopped. This is usually sufficient for the herb to improve an immune response against a cold or some other mild infection. Echinacea can be taken two times per day, for three to seven days, without side effects. Use it whenever you feel a cold coming on or when suffering from a cold or flu. The standard dosage is thirty drops of echinacea in tincture.

Ginseng

Ginseng *(Panax schinseng)* is a root with all sorts of powers claimed for it. One study showed that compounds within ginseng caused T lymphocytes to multiply more vigorously in response to a challenge. As with echinacea, however, higher levels of the same compounds inhibited proliferation. Volunteers given capsules containing one hundred milligrams of ginseng extract, twice a day for eight weeks, showed enhancement in a number of immune functions, including increased phagocytosis by macrophages and improved ability of granulocytes to kill foreign organisms.

Many products that are called ginseng do not come from *Panax* and probably lack the powers of real ginseng. Siberian and Brazilian ginseng come from different plant families and presumably have different effects, which currently are unknown. Ginseng is widely available in natural foods stores and Asian markets.

We recommend doses of one hundred milligrams, twice a day, for three to seven days, when the immune system needs boosting. Over several weeks, these doses will not cause harmful side effects and can boost immunity, but higher daily doses may inhibit the immune response.

Aloes

Several members of the Liliaceae family (which includes garlic) have been shown to enhance immune function. These include extracts of aloe plants such as *Aloe vera, Aloe barbadensis,* and *Paris formosana. Aloe vera* is a common plant and is widely used in the United States as a balm for all types of skin diseases and burns. Extracts from aloe are used in Southeast Asia to treat inflammatory diseases.

Aloe inhibits the release of oxidants by granulocytes without affecting their ability to phagocytize or kill microorganisms intracellularly. This prevents swelling of tissues, without decreasing the granulocytes' ability to destroy foreign organisms within the system.

A derivative of aloe (called Acemannan) has antitumor effects in animals and stimulates macrophages to make cancer-fighting cytokines, including interleukin-1 and tumor necrosis factor. A compound in *Paris formosana,* called formosanin C, increases the proliferation of lymphocytes and stimulates natural killer cell activity.

Aloe and its related plants are best used as topical ointments for burns, abrasions, skin disorders, and stings.

Astragalus

Astragalus is one of the most widely prescribed herbs in Chinese medicine and is available in natural foods stores and in many Asian markets. Extracts from astragalus have also been shown to boost immune response in people with normal immune systems, as well as those with impaired immunity.

In two studies, both controls and subjects with advanced cancer showed a two- to threefold increase in the strength of their immune response when a standard antigen skin test was administered. Proliferation of lymphocytes also increased, but less dramatically. Both these changes indicate improved cell-mediated immunity, meaning that T lymphocyte and macrophage activity was boosted.

A second study showed that astragalus boosted immune response even in animals that were treated with an immunosuppressive drug, cyclophosphamide.

To fight colds or flu, or as a boost to the immune system, astragalus can be added as an herb to soups and stews. Or you may add twenty to thirty drops of the herb tincture to water and drink it two times per day, for three days.

Green Tea and Black Tea

Both green and black teas contain antioxidants, bioflavonoids, tannins, and indoles, all of which are being demonstrated to fight cancer. Human population studies and animal research have shown a strong correlation between tea consumption and reduced risk of certain cancers, especially esophageal cancer. These teas, in regular or decaffeinated form, were also found to reduce the development of skin cancer in animal studies.

Green tea has been touted in the popular media as a protective agent against cancer, especially after it was learned that it is rich in antioxidants and that Japanese who drink green tea have lower rates of cancer. *The Lancet* reported recently that black tea contains just as many antioxidants as green tea, which means that it may well provide the same protection.

Tea contains about one quarter of the caffeine that coffee does.

Drink one or more cups of tea daily, or whenever desired.

Spices

Several spices have been shown to activate the immune system. These include saffron, ginger, clove, cumin, and turmeric. Use them in cooking whenever desired. The best approach is simply to flavor your foods with a wide variety of spices to make them delicious, satisfying, and health enhancing.

Saffron

Saffron has inhibited the growth of tumors in mice. It stimulated the proliferative response of T cells and elevated the levels of the antioxidant glutathione in the blood. Saffron therefore has an antioxidant effect.

Ginger

An extract of ginger *(Zingiber officinale)* has antifever and anti-inflammatory properties. Ginger is used as a tea and a condiment in Asian cuisine and for its healing properties in Chinese and Ayurvedic medicine. It has been shown to reduce the production of inflammation-causing prostaglandins and is also reported to reduce the pain of arthritis. Finally, ginger inhibits platelet aggregation, which means it improves blood circulation and offers some protection against heart attacks and strokes.

Turmeric

Turmeric, which is derived from the plant *Curcuma longa,* is widely used in Indian cooking and Ayurvedic medicine. It is anti-inflammatory and inhibits platelet aggregation. Research has shown that curcumin, a compound found in turmeric, is even more effective than beta-carotene in preventing the development of cancer in animals that have been fed a powerful carcinogen.

According to work done at M. D. Anderson Cancer Center in

Houston, turmeric inhibits cancer at several sites in the body by disrupting certain chemical processes that would otherwise lead to malignancy.

Turmeric has shown anti-HIV activity in the laboratory and is being tested currently in clinical trials.

Cumin

Cumin, from *Cuminum cyminum,* a very common spice, has been shown to inhibit platelet aggregation. Israeli scientists have found that people who regularly add cumin to their food have lower rates of urinary tract cancers, including those of the bladder and prostate. Scientists in India confirmed these findings and discovered that cumin greatly increased the body's production of a detoxifying agent, called GST, which inhibits cancer.

Clove

A substance derived from clove *(Syzygium aromaticum)* has demonstrated antitumor properties. The body maintains a balance between mature cells and immature cells by restricting the proliferation of immature cells; in cancer, immature cells that proliferate rapidly and actively are the most dangerous. Clove extract induced macrophages to target these immature cells more readily, thereby making them less of a threat.

Clove is not a healthful plant when used as an extract or in clove cigarettes. It can cause toxic reactions in the lungs, which have resulted in death when taken in high doses.

Promising New Research

A host of other plants traditionally used as herbs have been scientifically tested and shown to be significant immune system boosters. These herbs are widely available in natural foods and health food stores. Most come in easy-to-use tea bags or tinctures (add drops to water or fruit juice; use as directed on bottles). Some are spices that can be added to your cooking to enhance both the flavor and the healthfulness of a dish. The following herbs have just begun to gain scientific support for their health-enhancing powers.

- *Calendula officinalis,* commonly known as calendula, is available in dried form to be used as a tea or in tincture. It is an anti-inflammatory when applied topically.
- *Cassia garrettiana,* commonly known as senna, has traditionally been used as an intestinal cleanser. It inhibits histamine release in allergic reactions. It is widely available as a powder and as a fruit-based laxative.
- *Chamomilla recutita,* or simple chamomile, boosts phagocytosis. This herb is widely available in tea bags.
- *Plantago asiatica,* commonly known as plantain, has been used since the days of Hippocrates. It is available as a dried herb and in tincture. It stimulates phagocytosis and natural killer cell activity.
- *Tamarindus indica,* commonly known as tamarind, is widely used in India and in Indian cuisine as a fruit (from the tamarind tree) or as a medicinal herb, which comes from the leaves of the tree. It enhances phagocytosis and the trapping of white blood cells at inflammatory sites.

Special Foods That Fight Cancer

For people who are not familiar with traditional or herbal medicine, the word *herb* can conjure up images of strange foreign plants that have been specially prepared and then sprinkled into boiling water, perhaps with an incantation or two. Actually, traditional healers see herbs as nothing more than medicinal plants and not a form of magic. The more science learns about the healing agents available in the plant kingdom, the longer the list of medicinal plants becomes.

In fact, science is finding that the common foods you see at the market and on your plate contain remarkable immunity-boosting and cancer-fighting ingredients. A new array of cancer-fighting compounds has entered the scientific lexicon, including indoles, carotenoids, coumarins, bioflavonoids, isothiocyanates, phytochemicals, and sulforaphane, to name just a handful. These nutrients, discussed in the following pages, can make a difference in your health and your life.

The following foods contain cancer-protective nutrients. Place these vegetables on your menu often. While you enjoy their wonderful flavors, they will be protecting you against disease.

Cruciferous Vegetables

These green leafy vegetables (broccoli, cabbage, kale, brussels sprouts, collard and mustard greens, and watercress) contain compounds called phytochemicals and indoles that may prevent tumor-causing estrogen from targeting the breast. In animal studies, they've been shown to switch on enzymes that protect breast tissue from carcinogens. They are also rich sources of another cancer fighter called sulforaphane, a potent trigger for detoxifying tissues and blood and for promoting production of cancer-preventive enzymes.

Cruciferous vegetables, especially watercress, also contain a substance known as phenethyl isothiocyanate, which has been shown to inhibit the creation of lung tumors in animals injected with a powerful tobacco-derived carcinogen.

Soybeans and Soybean Products

Tofu, tempeh, miso, shoyu (soy sauce), and tamari are products made from soybeans that can be used in a variety of dishes.

Tempeh is a fermented soybean patty that can be sautéed or cut up and added to soups or stews. Miso, shoyu, and tamari are fermented soybean products. Miso is a soybean paste that has been fermented in salt from two months to two years. Often, a grain is added to the mix, such as wheat, brown rice, barley, or millet. Miso was created by the Japanese and used traditionally as a base for soups, stews, and sauces. Long a staple in Japan, miso soup is regarded by Japanese as a powerful healing food. Shoyu and tamari are two types of soy sauce, commonly used in Asia as a base for soups, stews, and sauces.

In April 1993, the *Proceedings of the National Academy of Sciences* reported that scientists had isolated a substance in miso and other soybean products that blocks blood flow to tumors, thus starving them from the essentials of life. The substance, called genistein, blocks blood vessels from growing into tumors, a process known as angiogenesis. Cancer cells and tumors, like all other cells and tissues in the body, need oxygen and nutrition to survive. In order for them to get both, they need blood. Thus, cancer is sustained within the body by blood vessels that grow to the cells and support their life. The genistein in miso soup blocks blood vessels from becoming attached to the cancer cells, and thus literally suffocates and starves the tumor.

Dr. Judah Folkmann of the Harvard Medical School, who has studied how blood vessels form to support the growth of cancerous tumors, said that genistein may be an ideal form of cancer therapy, one that attacks the cancer cells but leaves normal cells unaffected. Numerous studies by the Japanese National Cancer Center show that people who eat miso soup regularly have 33 percent fewer incidences of cancer than those who never eat it. Also, Dr. Wargovich has stated that soybeans contain a substance called protease inhibitor, which interferes with cancer cell proliferation at both the early and later stages of development.

Beans (Legumes)

Beans are the greatest source of protein in the vegetable kingdom. Collectively known as legumes, beans and peas generally contain between 20 and 30 percent protein. Rich sources of complex carbohydrates and fiber, they also contain significant amounts of vitamins and minerals. One hundred grams of soybeans, for example, contain 226 milligrams of calcium, 554 milligrams of phosphorus, 8.4 milligrams of iron, and 1,677 milligrams of potassium, according to the U.S. Department of Agriculture (USDA). One hundred grams of adzuki beans contain 21 milligrams of protein. One hundred grams of chickpeas contain 20 milligrams of protein, and the same amount of whole lentils contains 25 milligrams of protein, according to the USDA. All beans contain vitamins A and B, as well.

Like grains, beans contain soluble fibers that bind with fat and cholesterol and lower blood cholesterol levels. This prevents atherosclerosis, or cholesterol plaque that forms in the arteries to the heart and brain and causes heart attack and stroke.

But beans have other properties that scientists are just beginning to appreciate. The American Health Foundation reported that consumption of beans may well be the reason Hispanic women suffer such low rates of breast cancer. Hispanic women, who experience far lower rates of breast cancer than white women, eat a diet twice as rich in beans as white women. Upon further study, the researchers discovered that beans contain high amounts of an estrogen-blocking nutrient called phytoestrogen, which may protect against breast disease, including malignancies of the breast.

Fruit

Citrus fruits contain compounds called limonoids, which stimulate the production of protective enzymes. Most fruits contain bioflavonoids and antioxidants, which block the receptor sites for hormones that promote cancers.

■ ■ ■

Hippocrates put it well some twenty-five hundred years ago: "Let thy medicine be thy food and thy food be thy medicine." Today, after decades of dependence upon sophisticated drugs and an increasing pursuit of genetic treatments, the age-old wisdom of the "father of medicine" is still excellent advice.

CHAPTER EIGHT

Immune System Booster #5:
Exercise

Many of us have turned the old aphorism that exercise is good for us into a kind of hairshirt. We think that unless we engage in lots of exercise — that is, lots of sweat and pain — we won't get any benefit from it. Nothing could be further from the truth. From the point of view of the immune system, moderate exercise is ideal, which means that walking four times per week will boost immune system function and protect you from infection, cancer, and heart disease.

When viewed exclusively in terms of how it benefits the immune system, exercise presents a challenging paradox, however. On one hand, people clearly live longer and enjoy better health when they engage in regular, moderate exercise. Nevertheless, exercise is a stressor on the body, specifically on the immune system. Strenuous exercise depresses certain immune cell counts, at least temporarily. In addition, long-term exercise programs that are highly stressful, such as competitive long-distance running, result in consistently lower immunity, at least for certain immune factors.

Thus, contrary to what many people believe, there *is* such a thing as too much exercise. And like many other examples of "overdoing a good thing," too much exercise can weaken your immune response to disease-causing agents. Such revelations teach us, again, that balance is crucial to good health.

Interestingly, the effect of exercise on the immune system depends strongly on the degree of exertion, and hardly at all on the length of time spent exercising. For instance, thirty seconds of strenuous exercise causes changes in the relative numbers of white blood cells in the blood, whereas one hour of gentle exercise has no measurable effect on these cells. Also, the changes seen after thirty minutes of moderate exercise are the same as those seen after two hours of the same level of exercise.

Despite the fact that exercise has been studied so extensively, especially its impact on the cardiovascular system, there is still much to be learned about what exercise does for immune system function. In general, people who exercise moderately live longer and have lower rates of cancer and cardiovascular disease. Some or all of these benefits may be linked to the immune system. For example, moderate exercise boosts the function of macrophages, the cells that play a crucial role in the creation of atherosclerosis and heart disease. Recognizing this effect, some scientists have speculated that the benefits of exercise to macrophage cells may represent an independent protection against heart disease, quite apart from exercise's well-known benefits to heart function, circulation, and respiration. This and other questions have yet to be answered, however. What we do know is that *moderate* exercise has the best impact on the immune system.

The Immune System and Exercise: Some Good News, Some Bad

First the Good News

The effects of exercise on the immune system that have been studied most extensively are changes in the number and type of white blood cells, the ability of lymphocytes to proliferate, and the ability of natural killer cells to destroy target cells. In general, the number of all major classes of white blood cells — granulo-cytes, natural killer cells, monocytes (the circulating form of macrophages), and lymphocytes — increase during exercise, es-pecially if the exercise has not been highly strenuous.

Macrophages

Moderate exercise causes macrophages to more aggressively gobble up bacteria, viruses, and cancer cells. It also induces macrophages to produce more health-promoting cytokines, in-cluding interleukin-1 (which triggers inflammation), interleukin-6 (which is also proinflammatory), and tumor necrosis factor (which kills cancer cells and tumors).

In general, the research demonstrates that macrophages re-spond to exercise in ways that are very similar to their response to infection: they become more alert to and aggressive toward possible threats to health. Macrophages become particularly ac-tive in areas of inflammation, which may be one reason that exercise is associated with lower rates of cancer. Some studies have shown that macrophages enter muscle tissue and attack antigens after exercise.

Granulocytes

After a period of moderate exercise, granulocytes also are more aggressive in their consumption and destruction of antigens. They also show a marked improvement in their ability to target areas of the body where they may be needed and destroy foreign or invading bacteria or viruses.

Natural Killer Cells

Like macrophages and granulocytes, natural killer cells are more aggressive and more numerous after moderate exercise. Exercise appears to specifically promote the ability of natural killer cells to destroy tumors. This effect occurs even in elderly women who begin and consistently maintain exercise programs.

The immune changes induced by exercise tend to be short-lived. Most of the elevations or reductions in immune cells return to normal within fifteen minutes to two hours after exercising, although some last a day or more.

Now the Bad News

The ability of lymphocytes to proliferate, however, is suppressed after exercise. This weakening of immunity appears to be short-lived, however, and returns to normal within an hour or two. When T cells become sluggish, however, their ability to make cytokines, such as interleukin-2, is also reduced. That means that B cells become less responsive to antigens as well, since they depend on CD4 cells to order them to make antibodies.

The diminution of immune response after exercise appears to be strongest among competitive athletes who engage in highly demanding exercise regimes.

Overtraining and Immune Response

Exercise alters blood levels of certain stress hormones, such as cortisol, epinephrine, and beta-endorphin. The amount and types of hormones produced vary with the type of exercise and its degree of difficulty. The more strenuous the exercise, the more these stress hormones are created. Stress hormones, as we will see in Chapter 9, tend to weaken immune response.

One of the great benefits of exercise is that it pumps more oxygen into the blood, but here, too, there is a dark side to the benefit. As the cells respire, or breathe, they produce more oxidants, which break down molecules and form free radicals. This, in turn, raises the demand for certain antioxidants in the cells and bloodstream, especially for glutathione. The combination of hormonal changes, elevation of oxidants, and greater demand for antioxidants creates stresses on the immune system that, for the person on a poor diet, may well weaken overall immunity.

There is a well-known connection between overtraining in athletes and an increased susceptibility to infections. In studies comparing immune responses of highly trained athletes to those of control populations, the athletes came out the losers. Blood levels of lymphocytes, the blood and saliva levels of immunoglobulins, and the ratio of CD4 cells to CD8 cells were lower in the athletes than in the controls. Natural killer cell activity was also lower in the athletes.

The deleterious effects of overexercising are likely a combination of psychological and physical stress, coupled with a depletion of antioxidants in the bloodstream. While the German national field hockey team was preparing for the Olympic Games of 1988, the combination of intense exercise during workouts and the psychological stress of the approaching competition led to tremendous depressions of the players' immune systems. Some of the players had CD4 cell counts typical of AIDS patients.

Improving the nutrition of athletes seems to offset at least some of the negative effects of overtraining. One study showed that marathon runners who were given vitamin C after a race had lower rates of respiratory infections than those who were not given the vitamin, suggesting that replacing antioxidants helps buffer the negative effects of exercise. Other studies have supported the conclusion that, in addition to eating a highly nutritious diet, competitive athletes who undergo strenuous training should take antioxidants after vigorous exercise.

The Effects of Exercise on Illness

Cancer

Exercise appears to offer women significant protection against breast cancer. A recent study showed that exercise reduced the risk of breast cancer in Caucasian women forty years of age and younger, particularly those who had borne children. Women who exercised an average of at least forty-eight minutes per week were less likely to have developed cancer than those who exercised less or not at all. The greatest protection was seen in those who exercised the most, more than 3.8 hours per week.

Overall, there is a lower incidence of certain kinds of cancers in those who regularly exercise compared to those who do not.

Asthma and Allergies

For those who suffer from asthma and allergies, the best form of exercise seems to be yoga. Strenuous exercise, on the other hand, can cause problems.

Many studies indicate that exercise can precipitate an asthmatic episode and allergic reactions. The tendency to bring on such reactions may be due to the production of catecholamines (norepinephrine and epinephrine, both of which create excitation) during exercise.

Yoga appears to be an exception to this, causing no asthmatic or allergic reactions. In fact, at least one study has shown that yoga improved pulmonary function and reduced drug requirements for young asthmatics.

Arthritis

There are no ill effects, such as joint destruction, from exercise for patients with arthritis, according to research in which people with arthritis were followed for four years. A routine program of exercise is important for people with rheumatoid arthritis to increase cardiovascular strength, muscle endurance, and overall strength.

A study examining the effects of the Asian exercise tai chi chuan showed that the dancelike martial art caused no ill effects and was safe for people with rheumatoid arthritis.

Crohn's Disease

Exercise reduces the incidence of Crohn's disease, a form of inflammatory bowel disease. Those who exercise regularly have fewer flare-ups of the illness than those who do not.

Chronic Fatigue Syndrome

People with chronic fatigue syndrome who exercise moderately for thirty minutes per day show a decrease in fatigue, confusion, and depression.

Infections

Those who exercise moderately have the fewest infections, whereas those who engage in strenuous exercise, such as marathon runners, appear to have higher rates of infection, especially after a competitive event.

Stress and Emotional Problems

Exercise clearly boosts mood and relieves stress and depression. By elevating mood and increasing positive feelings about oneself and life in general, exercise indirectly enhances the function of the immune system.

A study published in *Postgraduate Medicine* (July 1990) reported that people who had formerly suffered from depression and other emotional problems experienced reductions in stress and anxiety and underwent fewer bouts of depression after they began exercising. Their capacity to deal with stress also increased with regular exercise. When stressful situations arose, they did not succumb to self-criticism and other kinds of negative thinking, habits of mind that existed before they had begun exercising. The researchers also found that consistent exercise seemed to bring about a type of emotional transformation. The people who participated in the study reported feeling healthier, emotionally brighter, and far more positive about life.

Such effects are not merely superficial changes of mood, but alterations in brain chemistry. The brain begins to produce beta-endorphins after only twenty minutes of running. Even chronic depression has been relieved by consistent exercise.

When it comes to relieving stress and boosting mood, aerobic exercise seems to have a greater impact than anaerobic exercises such as weight training. When the psychological effects of aerobic exercise were compared with those of weight training and no exercise at all, researchers found that aerobic exercise had the most elevating effect on mood and a sense of well-being.

Exercise, Aging, and Longevity

A study of elderly women showed that incidence of upper respiratory infections was lowest in those who exercised regularly, and especially low among the women who did regular calisthenics. Respiratory infections were highest among those who didn't exercise. Women whose only exercise was walking also benefited by having fewer respiratory infections; however, they did not have as low a rate of infection as those whose programs included regular calisthenics.

Not surprisingly, these immune improvements affect the quality of life, since people of any age who exercise regularly experience lower rates of chronic and degenerative diseases. Also, studies have shown that colds, bacterial infections, and flu viruses don't last as long in people who exercise regularly.

Scientists at the Institute for Aerobics Research and the Cooper Clinic in Dallas studied a group of 13,344 men and women for eight years to determine what effect, if any, exercise had on longevity. The scientists measured the subjects' fitness levels directly by having the people walk on a treadmill, rather than simply having them fill out questionnaires. The study participants were divided into five groups, according to their levels of fitness. The fitness groups ranged from those who lived sedentary lives to well-conditioned athletes. As expected, those who were most sedentary died the soonest. However, the scientists were surprised to find that the greatest health benefit was derived by those who simply got out and walked a half hour per day, three or four times a week. This small amount of exercise cut the risk of having a heart attack or cancer by more than half.

Other research has confirmed these findings. A study published in the *New England Journal of Medicine* (February 25, 1993) found that men who take up a vigorous sport between the ages of forty-five and fifty-four live, on the average, ten months longer than those who remain sedentary.

How Much Exercise Do You Need?

The overall impact of exercise on the immune system depends strongly on the degree of exertion and hardly at all on the length of time spent exercising. The changes seen after thirty minutes of moderate exercise are the same as those seen after two hours of the same exercise — once you reach your stride, your body tends to adapt and maintain its own balance.

To benefit from an aerobic program, you have to exercise for at least twenty minutes a day, three or four days a week. You must exercise at a rate that will raise your heart rate to 60 to 90 percent of its maximum, according to the American College of Sports Medicine. To avoid the immunity-suppressing effects of overtraining, 80 percent of maximum is a prudent goal.

To determine your maximum heart rate, subtract your age from 220. If you are 50 years old, your maximum heart rate would be 170. To benefit from an exercise session, a 50-year-old should achieve a heart rate of between 102 and 136 beats per minute and keep it there for 20 minutes.

Before you begin exercising, warm up by doing ten minutes of stretching exercises. If you choose to walk, begin at a pace slower than your optimal speed and gradually increase it to your exercising speed. This will prepare your heart, respiratory system, and muscles for your workout. When you have finished exercising, again do five to ten minutes of light stretching to cool down.

Very Important: Before you begin exercising, have your physician give you a complete checkup. Do not engage in competitive sports if you are out of shape and haven't been exercising for some time. People forget themselves in the heat of competition and overexert themselves, sometimes leading to heart attacks. Start slowly, and work your way toward a more demanding program.

An Immunity-Boosting Exercise Program

1. Pick a time during the day that you can exercise, and stick to that time. Most people enjoy exercising in the morning. You need only twenty to thirty minutes, during which you can walk around the block at least once, and, as you improve your fitness, more than once.

2. Exercise throughout the day. Walk the stairs, rather than taking the elevator. Walk to lunch, rather than grabbing a cab. Take a walk after lunch.

3. Enjoyment is the key. Pick an activity or a sport that you enjoy doing, and become really good at it. Popular exercises include walking, bicycle riding, tennis, swimming, water aerobics, and weight training at home.

4. Join the club. Membership in a YMCA, YWCA, or health club is a great way to work out and meet people. It takes care of at least two immune system boosters at once, since you'll be exercising and developing relationships at the same time. Many colleges and universities offer surprisingly inexpensive health and fitness programs.

5. Gadget lovers can buy an exercise machine, such as a stair-climbing machine, treadmill, cross-country ski equipment, a stationary cycle, or a Nautilus.

6. Turn a friend into an exercise partner. Sometimes having a partner can be just the incentive you need to keep going.

7. Dancing is aerobic, romantic, and social. There are lots of dance clubs — for contra dancing, square dancing, and swing — that provide lessons and social connections.

8. Join a nature and hiking club, another way to combine exercise with social needs. The added benefits are numerous: you get to be outdoors in nature, a big balancer of stress; you will learn about and become intimate with the natural world; and you'll gain the confidence that comes with such knowledge. The earth supports us, but only by spending time exploring the earth can we ever come to know this remarkable truth.

9. Adult education programs abound with exercise classes — everything from aerobics and stretching to tai chi chuan and the martial arts.

CHAPTER NINE

Immune System Booster #6:
Stress Reduction

THE SCENARIO IS ALL too familiar: you face a challenging situation, the outcome of which will have a dramatic impact on your life and perhaps on the lives of others. Responsibility for the success or failure of the venture falls heavily on your shoulders. You apply all your ability, you hope for the best, but you fear the worst. Meanwhile, dark possibilities about what *might* happen prey on your mind. You stay up late worrying about the many variables that may affect the outcome. Perhaps you lose some sleep. Physical symptoms arise: shortness of breath and nervous tension in your arms, hands, and stomach. Your heart races and may even palpitate; a pervasive feeling of confusion and doubt sets in. It's called stress. When it lingers for weeks or months, it's called chronic stress. It changes everything in your external environment and much of what goes on inside of you, as well.

The study of how stress affects your immune system, a science called psychoneuroimmunology, is among the most exciting areas of health research. Stress has a tremendous effect on the body's immune functions and the impact of stress on immunity demonstrates the power each of us has over our own health. By reducing or eliminating stress, you can remove a great burden from your immune system and thereby strengthen your immune response.

Most of us experience distress from time to time. Those of us who are chronically distressed, which means we are continually depressing our immune systems, are increasing our chances of becoming ill. Stress raises the likelihood that you will contract a bacterial infection and virus, including the common cold. It also increases your chances of suffering a serious degenerative disease, such as heart disease, high blood pressure, cancer, asthma, diabetes, and inflammatory bowel disease. Many physicians believe that stress plays a role in the onset of multiple sclerosis, rheumatoid arthritis, and other autoimmune diseases, though these links have yet to be proven. Nevertheless, science has shown that stress is clearly an immune system depressor, which means that it places us at risk for all kinds of disorders.

Stress and the Immune System

A variety of immune functions are influenced by stress. Recently, a team of researchers conducted a meta-analysis, or an overview of the best research in a specific field. After reviewing thirty-eight well-controlled studies examining the effects of stress on the immune system, the scientists concluded that stress consistently lowers several types of immune response. The immune system is simply weaker in people under stress.

People who are subjected to stress and then given an antigen are found to have lower immune responses than those who are not subjected to stress. In addition, natural killer cells decrease in number and activity in those under stress; in one study, changes in the cells' activity paralleled changes in adrenaline. The higher the adrenaline levels, the lower the natural killer cells' responses to a virus or cancer cell.

The research has also shown that the production of cytokines, such as interleukin-2 and gamma-interferon, also decreases under stress. This suggests that CD4 cells and macrophages are not functioning optimally (since they produce cytokines). The overall immune response will be weaker without such chemical messengers being sent out. Antibodies produced by B cells to fight herpes virus tend to be elevated when people with herpes are under stress. As we pointed out in Chapter 2, viruses such as herpes and HIV are capable of hiding within cells, where they remain dormant until the immune system is weakened, at which time the virus mounts an attack. The immune system responds in part by making antibodies to combat the virus. The struggle ensues. But the struggle occurred in large measure because the strength of the immune system dropped, which offered the virus an opportunity to come out of hiding, start replicating, and gain a greater foothold in the body.

A number of studies report that the ratio of CD4 cells to CD8 cells decreases, most often because the number of CD8 cells (the immune suppressors) increases.

Exams, Stress, and Immune System Depression

Ronald Glaser and Janice Kiecolt-Glaser, two longtime workers in the field of psychoneuroimmunology, have carried out a series of experiments over several years that examine the effects of exam stress on medical students at Ohio State University. Each year they look at immune responses of students during times of low stress and during the high-stress periods immediately before exams. Not surprisingly, the researchers found that exam stress is associated with a decrease in overall immunity. In addition, a number of specific immune responses were weakened, including T cell and natural killer cells and the production of interleukin-2 and gamma-interferon. The researchers also found an increase in Epstein-Barr virus antibodies, meaning that during high-stress periods, the virus had emerged from its hiding places within the tissues.

Other researchers have also documented changes in the immune response to common tasks such as arithmetic tests and stressful interviews, and in all of these experiments the observations were consistent: low natural killer cell activity and a low immune response to a challenge. The effect of stress on the immune system takes place quickly. Weakened immune responses were observed within thirty minutes of taking the test or undergoing the interview. Groups subjected to other stressful life events, such as parachuting or waiting for the result of an HIV test, experienced similarly impaired immune function.

Stress Has an Independent Effect

Skeptics argue that stress doesn't have an independent effect; rather, it encourages people to increase behaviors that are debilitating to the immune system, such as loss of sleep, poor eating, smoking, excessive drinking, and other health-impairing actions. This argument has been proved false, however.

Glaser and Kiecolt-Glaser considered other possibilities for immune system depression in students, such as lack of sleep or lack of eating, and found stress had an independent impact on immunity. When they looked at the effect of these factors independently, they found that changes in immune function did not correlate with sleep or weight changes, or with changes in blood protein levels that would indicate malnutrition. Stress was debilitating all by itself.

In another carefully controlled study, 154 men and 266 women were exposed to a virus and then monitored for the development of a cold. There was a striking linear correlation between the amount of stress reported by the subjects during the previous year and their susceptibility to colds. This study, as well as laboratory research, has offered convincing evidence that common stress-related behaviors are not the cause of observed changes in immune response.

Hormones and Stress

Stress, as many of us know firsthand, can wreak havoc with our hormones, which in turn can have profound effects on our health. Certain stress-related hormones contribute directly to cardiovascular disease. Some of these same hormones create immune system dysfunction, as well. Stress triggers the overproduction of a variety of neurochemicals. Among the most carefully studied of these is cortisol, a hormone produced by the adrenal glands. Cortisol prevents excessive use of energy in a crisis. It also inhibits almost all aspects of the immune system. Stress increases production of cortisol, which in turn reduces immune response across the board.

The catecholamines, which include epinephrine (also called adrenaline) and norepinephrine (a neurotransmitter that, like adrenaline, also gives rise to physical and emotional excitation), often cause the heightened physical sensations that we experience while under stress — fear, excess energy, rapid breathing and heart rate, and enhanced physical coordination. Depending on the quantity of such neurochemicals in the blood, they either enhance or interfere with the communication between an immune cell's receptors and the cell's nucleus. Unfortunately, whenever we are under stress — especially prolonged stress — these chemicals usually interfere with that communication, and thereby prevent immune cells from responding to antigens. Thus, hormonal imbalance weakens the immune response.

Aside from its effects on the immune system, stress is thought to contribute to the development of heart disease, asthma, ulcers, inflammatory bowel syndrome, diabetes, migraine headaches, and premenstrual syndrome.

Humans Versus Animals: We're Not the Better Adapters

Humans are far more vulnerable to long-term or chronic stress, the most debilitating kind, than are the other members of the animal kingdom. In animal studies, repeated exposure to stress, such as electrical shocks, causes the animal to adapt to the stress so that over time it loses its immunosuppressive effect.

However, in human studies the impairment of immune response tends to persist, especially when the source of the stress is interpersonal, which means it is not necessarily under a single person's control. Sometimes human responses to chronic stress can be maladaptive. For example, normally the body has a built-in monitoring system that can turn off further production of cortisol, an immunity-depressing hormone, whenever cortisol levels become too high. When chronic depression sets in, however, the monitoring system becomes inefficient so that cortisol continues to be overproduced.

Humans also show a marked propensity to become overly sensitized to stress so that even the mere suggestion of a particular stressor, like the bell in Pavlov's experiments, triggers a physical and, in this case, immunity-depressing response. For example, cancer patients who have undergone chemotherapy often suffer from nausea or vomiting whenever they anticipate or approach their next appointment for another round of drugs. Parallel changes occur in the immune system. Women with ovarian cancer, for example, were found to have reduced lymphocyte responses when their next chemotherapy appointment drew near.

This same phenomenon occurs in other settings in which people experience long-term stress. For example, those who care for victims of Alzheimer's and women who have recently suffered a divorce or who remain in unhappy marriages all show impaired immune responses. Specifically, natural killer cells are weakened, and, if the virus is present, herpes antibodies increase. Such conditions make people more susceptible to a wide variety of viral and bacterial diseases, as well as cancer.

Stress and Prenatal Considerations

Unfortunately, psychological stress during pregnancy can have long-lasting effects on offspring. The developing infant's brain is influenced by the abnormal levels of neurochemicals and hormones when the mother is under stress. Probably as a result of these changes during development, the immune response of the infant is weakened or impaired. Studies have shown that B cells and the antibodies they produce are particularly affected.

Eustress and Distress

Like beauty, stressful situations exist in the eye of the beholder. One person may perceive challenges at home or at work as opportunities — chances to make relationships better, to realize personal goals, and to utilize inherent abilities. This person is more likely to jump into the fray and, despite the difficulties, very often finds herself enjoying the process. She has a certain amount of freedom to express herself, to take risks, and to give herself latitude for experimentation and creativity. Hence, she becomes empowered in the face of difficulties and exercises a certain amount of control, which, as we will see in the next chapter, can enhance immunity. Conversely, another person perceives difficulties as a threat to her survival. She recoils from the challenge, plays it safe, and worries about the outcome of events. On some level, she realizes that she has little or no power over the situation because she has withdrawn from the challenge. This of course will affect the quality of her efforts — whether at home or at work — and undoubtedly will shape the outcome of events. More important, it will dramatically affect the quality of her life.

The first person is experiencing what scientists refer to as *eustress,* or the perception that within challenge lies opportunity. This perception is based on the belief that the outcome of the challenging situation very likely will be positive. Implicit within eustress are attitudes that support the immune system. The second person is experiencing *distress,* which is characterized by worry, anxiety, and fear. Distress arises from the belief that the outcome of the difficult situation will be negative. Distress depresses the immune system and can easily result in sickness.

Ironically, of two people facing the same situation, one can experience eustress while the other experiences distress. In other words, our attitudes often determine whether an event is challenging or distressing. Fortunately, our attitudes can change.

Science is learning that, with the help of an impressive array of techniques, you can transform your way of thinking and behaving to avoid the negative effects of stress. Not only can you alter the quality of your life — that has been known since the birth of religion — but such changes can dramatically boost your immune defenses. Here are some effective ways to do just that.

Mind Boosters to Boost Your Immune System

All of the following techniques help reduce stress and its negative side effects. Many of them not only prevent immune depression, but actually boost immune responses. However, some of the techniques we offer have not been specifically tested for their effects on immunity. But if we agree that excessive stress hurts the immune system (a well-established fact) and that reducing excess stress has a protective effect on immunity, it follows that the established techniques for relaxation and stress control will have, at the very least, a protective effect on the immune system.

Write Your Concerns in a Diary or Journal

Researchers in one well-known study asked students to write about upsetting events over a period of several days. Those that disclosed something that they had not previously talked about showed an improved immune response to mitogens. They also had fewer visits to the health clinic than their classmates. (See Chapter 11 for more on writing and confession.)

Pray, Meditate, or Repeat a Mantra

Nothing relaxes us like faith, and its effectiveness has been proved over and over again in the laboratory. Researchers at the University of Miami Medical School have found that daily meditation or relaxation exercises — that is, the progressive releasing of tension in muscles throughout the body — caused CD4 cells to increase. The study was done on men with HIV, who normally experience a steady decrease in CD4 cells. When Gail Ironson, M.D., a psychiatrist at the University of Miami Medical School, and her colleagues followed up on the men a year later, they found that those men who continued to do some form of daily meditation or relaxation exercises were less likely to suffer from AIDS symptoms.

Other research has shown that meditation or relaxation exercises have increased immune cell activity in the face of a challenge. One study showed an increase in natural killer cells and greater proliferation of lymphocytes in medical school students who practiced a daily relaxation regimen.

"There are many forms of relaxation or meditation exercises," says Dr. Ironson. "They can be as simple as muscle relaxation, or meditating on a beautiful place in nature, or repeating a single word (like a mantra) over and over again in your head. We don't have enough data to distinguish the effects of each of these practices on the immune system, but the research so far suggests that all of them — if practiced regularly — seem to have a positive effect."

Harvard University psychologist Ellen Langer found that transcendental meditation (TM) — a technique in which a person silently repeats a word, or mantra, over and over again — induces a deep state of relaxation and may be associated with increased longevity. After three years of study, Langer found that nursing home residents who practiced TM lived longer than those who didn't use the technique. All of the nursing home residents who practiced TM were still alive after three years of study, compared to a 38 percent death rate among patients who didn't use the technique.

Herbert Benson, M.D., associate professor of medicine at Harvard Medical School, has extensively studied the effects of prayer and meditation on health and found that such methods create what Benson calls the "relaxation response." A ten- to twenty-minute session of meditation per day, Benson says, lowers blood pressure, slows heart rate, relaxes muscles, and creates a more balanced hormonal condition, which all can contribute to a stronger immune response.

Use a Progressive Relaxation Technique

Like meditation, progressive relaxation techniques can change hormonal levels, causing a decrease in the immunosuppressive hormone cortisol while increasing the immunity-enhancing hormone dehydroepiandrosterone sulfate. One study found that relaxation training increased the overall immune response in nursing home patients. Another experiment found that relaxation triggered increased natural killer cell activity and the proliferation of lymphocytes in medical students undergoing examinations, ordinarily a situation that depresses the immune system.

One study found that the combined effects of relaxation techniques, exercise, and stress management increased T cells by 10 percent in a group of men infected with HIV. Another study reported that relaxation techniques, when combined with dietary change and mild exercise, were just as effective at lowering blood pressure as drug treatment, except that behavioral change had the added benefit of improving energy and sexual satisfaction.

Meditate

Chapters 9 and 10 contain suggestions for meditating. Try meditating twice a day to relieve stress and deepen spirituality. The following meditation is an example of a progressive relaxation technique that has been used with success by many people.

Lie comfortably on your back. Breathe rhythmically and deeply in a relaxed manner. Visualize your feet. Tense your toes and feet, and then suddenly relax them. Do the same with your calves: visualize the muscles of your calves, tense them, and then suddenly relax them. Do the same in sequence for your thighs, buttocks, stomach, chest, shoulders, hands, forearms, biceps, neck, and face. This meditation will create deep relaxation, and relieve muscle tension and stress.

Do some variation on this exercise daily and whenever you are under stress.

Try Biofeedback

Biofeedback may be the most effective technique for teaching people to achieve deep relaxation and to control tension and stress-related symptoms. Essentially, the states of deep relaxation created during biofeedback sessions are the same as those experienced in meditation and progressive relaxation. The only difference is that you achieve such conditions with the help of technological devices that measure body temperature, perspiration, heart rate, and other physical symptoms. People learn to control all of these physical symptoms with the use of such equipment. They see firsthand that they can lower their temperature, perspiration, and heart rate with their minds, and in the process they achieve deep relaxation and enhanced immunity.

Biofeedback has proved effective in the treatment of a wide range of problems, including angina, anxiety, asthma, intestinal disorders, chronic pain, epilepsy, headaches and migraines, high blood pressure, high cholesterol, insomnia, learning disabilities, muscle spasm, phobias, rapid heart rate, TMJ (temporomandibular joint dysfunction), and urinary problems.

Join a Support Group

Structured groups can focus on education, social support, relaxation training, or development of coping skills. At least two studies show improvement of immune system function in people involved in support groups. In one study, group support for melanoma patients resulted in reductions in anxiety and depression and a parallel boosting of immune response. Natural killer cell activity was particularly enhanced. So, too, were survival rates. Support groups have also been shown to increase longevity for people suffering from cancer, especially women with breast cancer.

Laugh More

It's no joke. A hearty laugh has been shown to increase IgA (immunoglobulin A), a virus fighter. A simple smile changes brain chemistry, relaxes muscles, and boosts immunity. It also triggers the production of endorphins, the opiate-like chemicals that provide feelings of well-being and the so-called natural high. Laughter causes temporary muscle contraction and then release, inducing deeper relaxation and lower blood pressure. Research at the University of California at Santa Barbara found that laughter was just as effective at reducing stress as biofeedback training. Scientists are finding that even changing your facial expression from a frown to a smile directly alters mood for the better. Researchers at Clark University in Worcester, Massachusetts, found that simply having people adopt the facial expression of a particular mood actually created that mood in the people themselves. Expressions of fear brought on feelings of fear and stress. The same consistency of feeling and expression occurred when the study's subjects were asked to adopt expressions of anger, disgust, and sadness. Conversely, when researchers asked people to repeat over and over again the letter *e,* which makes the face adopt an expression similar to a smile, feelings of happiness were engendered.

This research supports the old ditty that urges us to "spread sunshine all over the place, and put on a happy face." Nothing takes the tension out of a difficult situation better than humor. Wise people cultivate humor as a way of coping with life because — let's face it — a lot of life is absurd.

Consider Therapy

Seek out a professional counselor who can help you express your feelings and develop new ways to deal with difficult situations. Expressions of pain or anger, by themselves, have not been shown to improve mood or immune response. However, patients in therapy who are encouraged to express pain and anger while at the same time learning new life-supportive behaviors have shown significant improvement in mood.

Take a Warm Bath

Believe it or not, warm baths cause more than a placebo effect. Warm water relaxes muscles, improves circulation, and slightly warms the brain, which scientists say is calming to the entire system. The water temperature should not exceed 102 degrees Fahrenheit. Excess heat can be shocking to the system, causing muscles to contract while increasing circulation — an unhealthy combination. Soak in the tub for no more than fifteen minutes. (People with diabetes should entirely avoid hot baths.)

Breathe Deeply

Dean Ornish, M.D., director of the Preventive Medicine Research Institute in Sausalito, California, says that "deep breathing is one of the simplest, yet most effective stress-management techniques there is." Ornish demonstrated reversal of atherosclerosis in the coronary arteries — a historic step in medicine — by using a program that included a low-fat diet, mild exercise, and stress management. Ornish's stress management program was centered primarily on deep breathing — especially to relieve physical tension — and yoga. Deep and lasting exhalation is particularly relaxing. It releases physical tension and creates a centered feeling that is remarkably free of tension.

Consider Bodywork

Bodywork, such as acupressure, massage therapy, and therapeutic touch, creates profound relaxation and positively affects biochemistry and some immune responses. Make sure you see a certified professional.

Try Hypnosis

Like relaxation techniques, hypnosis can induce deep relaxation and improved biochemical conditions. If none of the other relaxation techniques appeal to you, try hypnosis.

Exercise the Blues Away

Studies show that people who exercise enjoy improved psychological health and greater self-esteem than those who don't. Exercise boosts mood and reduces depression, anxiety, and stress. It can even create euphoria. It also lowers blood pressure, elevates HDL (the type of cholesterol that protects against atherosclerosis), and strengthens cardiovascular function. (See Chapter 8 for more on exercise and the mind.)

Exercise changes brain chemistry. Twenty minutes of running causes the brain to secrete beta-endorphins, which relieve depression and create feelings of well-being and optimism. Studies have shown that running can be just as effective at enhancing one's psychological state as certain psychotherapeutic techniques. One study that examined the effects of exercise on people in a psychiatric hospital unit found that exercise significantly decreased depression and anxiety, and increased a sense of accomplishment. Dr. Dorothy Harris, a sports psychologist and professor at Pennsylvania State University, says that running for twenty minutes, three times per week, can have a profound effect on mental attitude and health.

Eat for Your Mind As Well As Your Body

Every meal changes brain chemistry and mood, according to research conducted at the Massachusetts Institute of Technology. Researcher John D. Fernstrom, Ph.D., has written that "it is becoming increasingly clear that brain chemistry and function can be influenced by a single meal. That is, in well-nourished individuals consuming normal amounts of food, short-term changes in food composition can rapidly affect brain function."

According to MIT researchers, carbohydrates found in whole grains and whole grain breads stimulate the production of a chemical neurotransmitter called serotonin, which creates feelings of well-being and inner peace. Serotonin calms anxiety, focuses the mind, alleviates depression, and produces sounder sleep. As carbohydrate intake increases, serotonin levels rise, along with all of these positive emotions.

According to Judith J. Wurtman, Ph.D., another of the MIT scientists and a pioneer in this field, "Those who eat calming foods [containing carbohydrates] report feeling more relaxed, more focused, less stressed, less distracted after their meal." Indeed, after people eat carbohydrates they report that "feelings of stress and tension are eased and the ability to concentrate is enhanced," says Dr. Wurtman.

On the other hand, scientists have found that meals rich in animal protein cause an increase in dopamine and norepinephrine, two neurotransmitters that increase alertness, responsiveness, and aggression. The more protein you eat, the lower your serotonin levels will be. Hence, protein foods elevate neurotransmitters that compete with, and ultimately lower, brain levels of serotonin.

■ ■ ■

Whichever stress-reduction techniques you incorporate into your lifestyle, you can rest assured that you will benefit both your state of mind and the fitness of your immune system.

CHAPTER TEN

Immune System Booster #7:
Beliefs and Attitudes That Heal

ALL OF US WOULD AGREE that beliefs and attitudes are part of what shapes our lives. They are the filter through which we judge experience to be either good or bad, life-supporting or threatening. Indeed, beliefs and attitudes are usually the most important factor in determining whether or not we experience stress, and how debilitating that stress will be to our immune systems.

Beliefs and attitudes, like so much else within the emotional realm, are elusive entities, difficult to articulate and even harder to understand — even when they are our own. What are your core beliefs? Why do you have them? How do they shape your perception of reality? Are you an optimist or a pessimist? Are you sure you know? Such self-knowledge is needed in order to make use of the information that follows.

Commenting on core beliefs, Albert Einstein went right to the center of things (as he so often did). He presented a simple question that can clarify our basic attitudes about life. "The most important question all of us must answer," he said, "is whether the universe is a friendly place or not."

Though the question can be answered with elaborate explanations — or evasions — each person's response can ultimately be boiled down to a simple yes or no. And from your one-word response flow most of your attitudes toward life, and indeed, your answer helps determine the condition of your immune system.

If you truly believe that the universe is a friendly place, you will be able to relax and feel optimistic about what to expect, say, in the next ten minutes and in the next ten years. You expect the universe to present you with much that is good, life-supporting, and even beautiful. This is what it means to be optimistic about life and the future, and this attitude will have a very powerful and very positive effect on your health.

This is not to say that optimistic people are Pollyannas or fools. Virtually all optimists would acknowledge that bad things happen in life and that everyone suffers. Still, an optimist believes that the universe is essentially good, even though he or she doesn't always understand why life unfolds as it does.

One of the interesting things about optimists is that they answer Einstein's question from their own *experience* of life. That is, they answer the question on the basis of how they assess their own lives, rather than how they intellectually judge the world at large. Part of the world might be heading straight into hell with alacrity, but the optimist believes that she has had more good fortune than bad, and that her future will be much the same.

Optimism has a strange power to influence how we affect other people. A person with a generally positive attitude toward life has a certain buoyancy. He is able to be a little more tolerant or generous in the moment, which means he tends to elicit the better parts of people and situations without really trying.

Optimism has other curious effects, especially on the optimist himself. It leads the optimist to feelings of gratitude and the desire to share his good fortune with others. In short, optimism tends to inspire actions that are benign and just plain helpful to others. The person who sends out a positive message very often gets a positive response. Hence, optimism is a kind of self-fulfilling prophecy, as Norman Vincent Peale noted more than four decades ago.

On the other hand, those who say that the universe is not a friendly place are continually on the alert for the moment when the universe — in the form of an unexpected event — rears up and commits some kind of crime against them. They expect the worst. Hence, pessimists tend to focus on bad things that have happened to them and to other people. They reason that this state of affairs exists because the universe is chaotic or downright unjust; consequently, evil prevails.

Because of actual negative experiences, many people have good reason for holding such an attitude. Indeed, evidence in support of pessimism is everywhere. But that's the trouble with reality: it tends to be so rich, so complex, and so thoroughly paradoxical that you can find just about anything you want to find to prove a given point. Indeed, many people argue that you can elicit anything you want, or expect, from most situations in life.

Nobody is an objective witness to reality. Objectivity doesn't even happen in the laboratory, as quantum mechanics has proved. As Heisenberg's uncertainty principle has taught us, observers tend to see those events that support their existing beliefs. Therefore, the person who has a pessimistic view of life focuses on events — or the facts within events — that support his attitudes and beliefs. Like optimism, pessimism is also self-fulfilling.

The existence of this tendency is borne out by research. A recent study reported in *The Lancet* (November 1993) found that people who, early in life, came to believe they were predisposed to life-threatening illnesses actually died sooner than those who did not share such beliefs. Researchers followed Chinese Americans who were born during certain years that they believed predisposed them to lethal diseases. They actually died four years sooner, on average, than Chinese Americans born during other years, and at least four years sooner than white Americans who actually had the same diseases as the Chinese Americans but held more positive beliefs about the outcomes of those illnesses. The findings were based on a very large sampling — 28,169 Chinese Americans and 412,632 white Americans. Study leader David P. Phillips, Ph.D., professor of sociology at the University of California at San Diego, feels that this study suggests that beliefs can have a dramatic effect on health. "Our findings and those of others suggest that mental attitude is associated with health," he says.

Pessimism inevitably leads to hostility, often directed against oneself. It also leads to certain behaviors that can be characterized as punishment or revenge. Of course, people do not necessarily see their actions as revenge; they may see them as a form of justice. The act itself is referred to as "getting even," "punishing the guilty," or "seeking vengeance for a wrong." Revenge may be no more malicious than the feeling that something has been taken from you — love or attention, perhaps — and you want to rectify that in some way. It can be as subtle as withholding love (sometimes that is the only power a person feels he has) or as overt as an act of violence.

In his book *The Stress of Life* (1956), pioneer stress researcher Dr. Hans Selye recognized gratitude and revenge as the two most significant attitudes for determining the quality of one's existence. Indeed, Selye maintained that these two attitudes determine whether or not a person experiences deep and abiding stress, or is healthy and capable of enjoying life. As he put it, "It seems to me that, among all the emotions, there is one which, more than any other, accounts for the absence or presence of stress in human relations: that is the feeling of gratitude — with its negative counterpart, the need for revenge. I think in the final analysis that gratitude and revenge are the most important factors governing our actions in everyday life."

That insight goes to the very heart of human nature. Indeed, it penetrates to the essence of motive and to the very foundation of our attitudes. Gratitude and revenge, optimism and hostility create different internal conditions and have very different effects on health.

■ ■ ■

When people talk about attitudes and beliefs that form the foundation of our lives and thus determine the level of stress in daily life, they are discussing our relationship with the universe and have entered into the spiritual dimension of life, where the deepest and most significant questions and answers lie. This most personal of all realms offers perhaps the greatest possibilities for transformation. The authors of this book do not intend to provide answers to questions of the spirit. Rather, we wish to direct readers within, so that they might better understand — and perhaps improve — their own attitudes. We will show that positive attitudes have positive effects on immunity, whereas negative attitudes are debilitating to health. But if we do not first seek to understand our attitudes and their roots, such information may be useless. Honest soul searching and the willingness to change are both important.

Feeling "in Control": An Immune System Booster

Attitude can make the difference between the suppression or boosting of the immune system. Researchers are now discovering that there is a direct link between the nervous and immune systems. Immune cells have receptors for chemicals produced by the brain, chemicals that are associated with specific moods. Thus, a biochemical link exists between emotions and immunity.

The feeling that you are in control of a situation actually boosts the immune system. In fact, a sense of mastery allows us the safety to interpret otherwise stressful situations as exciting and challenging. The seminal experiment that demonstrated this dynamic was done by Mark Laudenslager and colleagues at the University of Colorado. The researchers took a pair of rats and placed them in separate adjacent cages. The cages were wired to give each rat an identical electric shock. The difference between the two cages was that only one allowed the rat to control the shocks; the rat did this by turning a wheel within the cage. By doing this, the one rat could end the shocks to both cages. This meant that both rats were shocked for exactly the same duration. The only difference was that one rat had control over the shocks, and the other didn't.

Despite the fact that both rats were equally shocked by the current, only the helpless rat had a lowered immune response to a mitogen. (A mitogen is a substance that stimulates lymphocytes to divide.) The rat who could control the shocks experienced insignificant changes in its immune response. This study showed that a sense of helplessness, or the lack of control, influences how the body responds to stress.

A variation of this experiment was recently conducted with people, using noise as the stressor. One group could end the intermittent noise by pressing a control button in a pattern they had to figure out. A second group was told to sit and endure the noise. A third group was told that they could turn off the noise when they figured out the button sequence — as the first group had been told — but this instruction was false. No matter what sequence they pushed buttons in, they could not shut off the noise. Nevertheless, they continued to try to stop the noise, demonstrating that they believed they had the power to stop it, despite the evidence to the contrary. The study took place over seventy-two hours, and the results of the study were most interesting.

The first group replicated the rat data: those who had the

power to control the noise had insignificant declines in their immune response, including activity of natural killer cells. For the most part, their immune systems remained strong. Those who lacked the power to control the noise showed a decrease in immunity, especially in natural killer cell activity. Remarkably, the last group had virtually the same results as the first: they, too, experienced little or no decline in immune function. The authors interpreted the results to show the importance of perceiving that you are in control, even when you aren't.

Depression and the Immune System

Certainly, the opposite of feeling in control is a sense of helplessness, which can lead to depression. A number of studies have shown that depression is associated with declines in immune responses. The older and more depressed a person is, the more severe is the immunosuppression, which most often includes low natural killer cell activity and low overall immune response to mitogens. The results are the same for major depression and a less serious chronically depressed mood.

Michael Irwin, a psychiatrist at the San Diego Veterans Center, studied women whose husbands were terminally ill with lung cancer or had recently died. He found that bereavement, of itself, did not depress natural killer cells, but those women who were more depressed had low natural killer cell activity.

Depression and Hormones

Depression is associated with higher than normal levels of cortisol, a hormone that suppresses immune response. Some depressed patients also show abnormalities in the catecholamines. Abnormal levels of catecholamines (such as adrenaline) may cause low natural killer cell activity.

Depression and Cancer

There is conflicting data on whether depression is associated with higher rates of cancer. Recently, a meta-analysis of the existing research was conducted in an attempt to see what, if any, overall pattern existed. The analysis showed that a marginally significant increase in cancer exists among depressed people. The cumulative data suggest that the difference in cancer incidence between those who are depressed and those who aren't is between 1 and 2 percent.

Although evidence linking depression as a contributor to cancer is weak, a growing number of studies suggest that attitude strongly affects the outcome of disease, including cancer, after it appears.

Optimism and the Immune System

Recently, researchers from the University of Pittsburgh Medical School, Yale University, and the Pittsburgh Cancer Institute together conducted a study of cancer patients who took relaxation and cognitive therapy designed to boost optimism and overcome self-defeating beliefs. The patients, thirty in all, suffered from a type of cancer that had an extremely high likelihood of recurrence. "The course was designed to make them more optimistic about events in their lives; it didn't focus on cancer," says Martin Seligman, a psychologist at the University of Pennsylvania who participated in the study.

Remarkably, the course worked: it did indeed make the participants more optimistic, which in turn resulted in a marked improvement in immune system function. The scientists discovered that the patients who took the course had more natural killer cells than the control group, which was made up of patients who received only the standard medical treatment. Natural killer cells are one of the most important immune system constituents in the body's fight against cancer because they target and destroy tumors and cancer cells.

The research on the effects of optimism and pessimism reveals a rippling effect that extends throughout our lives. Dr. Seligman and his colleagues surveyed sales representatives at the Metropolitan Life Insurance Company and found that the positive thinkers among the longtime staff sold 37 percent more insurance than did the pessimists. Of the newly hired workforce, the optimists outsold the pessimists by 20 percent. When Seligman and his colleagues examined the attitudes of the two groups, they found that the optimists tended to blame their failures on external events, such as the weather, the phone connection, or the fact that the customer was in a bad mood that day. Optimists also tend to vary their routines. If one approach did not work, they had the resilience to try another. Finally, when the optimist succeeded, she took the credit and congratulated herself. The pessimist, on the other hand, tended to blame herself for her failures and saw her successes as a fluke. Pessimists were quicker to give up, as well.

Optimism and Feeling "in Control"

As we saw earlier, one of the keys to a healthy immune system is a sense of control. Craig A. Anderson, a psychologist at Rice University in Houston, says that optimists tend to feel more in control of their circumstances than pessimists do. If events go badly for an optimist, he usually creates a new approach or strategy, believing that if he persists, the events will turn in his direction. The pessimist, says Anderson, feels cursed by fate (or, to put it another way, he feels that the universe is unfriendly). He perceives himself as helpless and therefore gives up sooner.

As a practical matter, optimists have the better chance at success, since repeated effort raises the odds in their favor. But behavior based upon optimism is obviously more self-empowering, since it includes an implicit belief that one's efforts will eventually pay off.

After studying women with advanced breast cancer, Dr. Sandra Levy of the Pittsburgh Cancer Institute found that women who were generally optimistic experienced longer periods of being disease-free, the best predictor of survival. On the other hand, the disease recurred sooner among the pessimists.

Dr. Christopher Peterson of the University of Michigan has found that pessimists tend to have poorer health habits, are more likely to indulge in high-fat foods, are more likely to drink excessively, and do not exercise as much as optimists. As we have already seen in other chapters, these behaviors depress the immune system.

Ultimately, optimism is the key to feeling in control and successfully handling stressful situations.

Anger

Anger is acutely stressful and can be physically debilitating, especially to the cardiovascular system. A growing body of evidence is demonstrating that hostile people suffer heart disease sooner than people who are more peaceful. Researchers at Stanford University discovered that bursts of anger can reduce the heart's pumping ability by as much as 5 percent. Although 5 percent does not seem like a great deal, cardiologists say that such a drop in the heart's efficiency for people who already suffer from heart disease can be extremely dangerous. Redford Williams, M.D., director of Behavioral Medicine Research Center at Duke University Medical School, told *The New York Times* that "with this magnitude of decrease in cardiac efficiency, all kinds of bad things can happen: a clot can form, ischemia can set the stage for a potentially fatal arrhythmia."

Becoming More Optimistic, Less Angry, and More Upbeat

Here are four steps that can help you develop greater optimism and a far greater sense of safety.

1. Consider Einstein's question, your answer to it, and how that answer might affect the rest of your life. If your approach to life thus far has been pessimistic, open yourself up to letting go of old attitudes and adopting new ones, especially in light of the proven effects of optimism on health, personal relationships, and professional life.

2. For many people, this effort will mean joining (or rejoining) a church, synagogue, or temple, or embarking on a search for a meaningful spiritual life. For others, it will mean adopting a program of prayer, meditation, chanting, or some other form of spiritual practice. First, you may need to confront your grief, disappointment, and sense of injustice concerning your life so far; you may need to make peace with your inner self and your concept of a supreme being.

   For those who wish to establish a spiritual meditative practice, the first thing to do is to create a peaceful and even sacred place in your home. Find a corner or a room that is not part of the day's routine traffic. You might create an altar or shrine. Include a special book (the Bible, the Tao Teh Ching, the Bhagavad Gita, or one of the Sutras of the Buddha, for example), various spiritual symbols or stones, and perhaps pictures or photographs of important relatives, friends, or teachers. Add candles or incense, if you like. Let this place become the external symbol of some peaceful place within your spirit. Each day, go to this place, and meditate and pray. With time and consistent practice, this place can become very powerful in your life. It is a safe haven, a place to go whenever you feel fear, anger, or conflict, or need special assistance. It can be a spiritual refuge.

You might go to this place each morning and evening of every day. Spend as little as ten minutes or as long as you like. Choose spiritual meditations from your own tradition or from some other path that you feel connected to, or invent your own.

- Meditation and prayer are powerful tools that work in mysterious ways. Frequently, they open us up to new possibilities and greater awareness, which can become the basis for greater freedom and a sense of rebirth.

- As psychotherapist and mind-body expert Jon Kabat-Zinn told television reporter Bill Moyers, "Emotions are not bad — they're just what you're feeling. The point is to get out of the same emotional ruts. Meditation can wake you up to the fact that in the present moment there may be new options and new ways of relating to old situations. We've found people who were very dissatisfied in their relationships with their bosses or their spouses or children, who were able to encounter these people in a totally new way. Even if a lot of negativity is coming at them, they can learn to breathe with it and find a new kind of response that completely changes the ground on which everybody's standing."

3. Make positive connections to people in the following ways:
   - *As healers.* Consult a truly understanding and healing physician, counselor, psychotherapist, or alternative healer who can help you heal physical, psychological, or spiritual wounds. Among the best alternative healing programs are acupuncture; acupressure and various other forms of bodywork, such as therapeutic massage; and therapeutic touch or

the laying on of hands. Ask friends and your physician for references for trusted professionals.

- *As a member of a community of like-minded people.* This can take place in a religious community, a support group composed of people dealing with issues similar to your own, or a therapeutic group. You might choose a men's support group or a women's support group; a twelve-step program, such as Alcoholics Anonymous; a group dedicated to supporting people with specific illnesses or histories of abuse; a naturalist society; a music group; a book club; a service club, such as the Lions, the Rotary, the Knights of Columbus, or a veterans' organization. Join a group that helps improve other people's lives (soup kitchens, the Salvation Army, Big Brothers/Big Sisters, or others).

- *As friends.* Become committed to one-on-one relationships in which intimacy and personal contact thrive. (See Chapter 11 for more on intimacy and healing.) Friendships can develop in your religious or support community, clubs, or other social avenues.

4. Keep a journal, and write down your reasons for feeling disappointment, sadness, injustice, anger, rage, and whatever other dark and hidden feelings may be wounding you inside. Then write down what you intend to do with these feelings that will heal them.

Dr. Redford Williams of Duke University Medical School offers the following seventeen points for healing hostility:

1. Reason with yourself.
2. Stop hostile thoughts, feelings, and urges.
3. Distract yourself.
4. Meditate.

5. Avoid overstimulation.

6. Assert yourself.

7. Care for a pet.

8. Listen!

9. Practice trusting others.

10. Take on community service.

11. Increase your empathy.

12. Be tolerant.

13. Forgive.

14. Have a confidant.

15. Laugh at yourself.

16. Become more religious.

17. Pretend today is your last.

Choose the strategies that appeal to you and work best for you. The goals of conquering pessimism and restoring optimism are what really matters. The way is up to you. In the end, the transformation that you undergo will improve the quality of your life, and perhaps even the quantity. As Dr. Phillips says, "In many ways, you have a greater ability to affect your longevity than your physician does."

CHAPTER ELEVEN

Immune System Booster #8:
Intimacy and Relationships

ANYONE WHO DOUBTS THAT we are social beings, biologically and psychologically in need of one another, should look at the medical literature linking immune response to supportive relationships. Married people tend to have stronger immune systems than the unmarried, just as happily married people have more vigorous immune responses than the unhappily married. In virtually every aspect of life, harmonious relationships — including the relationship with the self — usually result in better health.

Being truly alone, without connection to others, ironically causes us to be less connected to ourselves. We seek out relationships for many reasons, but in every one of them we demand the same thing: to be recognized and loved for our uniqueness, while at the same time wanting desperately to love and feel connected to another. And in this pull and push, we somehow manage to find ourselves and our place in the grand bazaar of the human community.

Needless to say, this is the challenge of challenges, but for those who manage it — or at least find some semblance of this balance — there is the reward of better physical, psychological, and spiritual health, which is the basis for a stronger immune response.

Intimacy Begins with You: Knowing Yourself

Before you can feel truly in touch with others, you must feel truly connected to yourself, lest you get lost in the demands and swirling winds of relationship. Being connected with your own inner self is one of the more difficult tasks of life, especially if you have suffered from a traumatic event. Yet the research shows that people who reconnect with themselves by confessing their secret pain have a stronger immune response to external antagonists.

This remarkable insight was discovered by James W. Pennebaker, Ph.D., a professor of psychology at Southern Methodist University in Dallas, Texas. After finding that writing about his own secret pain helped him recover from depression, Pennebaker devised a study in which people were to write for twenty minutes a day, for four consecutive days, about their most traumatic life event. He and other researchers — notably Janice Kiecolt-Glaser and Ronald Glaser — then measured the immune response of the participants and compared them against a control group. Time after time, the people who wrote in their journals about their own traumatic experiences had stronger immune responses.

There was a certain rule that had to be observed, however. The participants had to write about specific traumatic events in their lives, events that were never talked about with other people or that contained information that was never shared before. It was particularly important to write about the pain, anger, remorse, and guilt they may have felt regarding the event.

After the writing exercise, Pennebaker tested the number and responsiveness of T cells in both the control group and in those who spent four days writing confessional journals. He discovered that the T cells of students who did the writing were more proliferative in response to a mitogen than those of the control group. The students who kept journals had fewer visits to the health clinic than their matched controls. The immune response was especially strong among those people who confessed feelings that they had never confronted, even to themselves. These people, whom Pennebaker termed "high disclosers," had the most remarkable improvement in T cell response of all participants.

Pennebaker maintains that more than mere catharsis is at work here. He suggests that psychological inhibition — the mechanism by which we keep things secret, even from ourselves — requires a certain degree of psychic and physical energy. As he puts it, inhibition is a demanding form of work, especially when a very painful trauma must be kept secret. Physical symptoms frequently occur as a result of such inhibition, such as elevations in blood pressure, heart rate, breathing, skin temperature, and perspiration levels.

Pennebaker notes that these same symptoms occur when crime suspects undergo polygraph, or lie detector, tests. After working with polygraph experts at the Federal Bureau of Investigation, Pennebaker found that when suspects confess their crime and undergo subsequent polygraphs, they are remarkably relaxed and all their physical symptoms related to inhibition disappear.

The release that accompanies confession, therefore, occurs on both psychological and physical levels. Pennebaker even found that when criminals confess during polygraph tests, they often feel bonded to their confessors; many send them Christmas cards and letters, thanking them for their help. In effect, some correction of an imbalance has occurred that releases energy and restores psychic equilibrium. With this restoration of balance come feelings of peace, tranquillity, and resolution, as well as better health.

This same phenomenon occurs in people who use the writing method, or what has come to be known as the "Pennebaker method." During the first two days of writing, people experience negative emotions, such as anger, sadness, anxiety, and grief. On the third or fourth day, however, they experience feelings of relief, insight, and resolution.

Pennebaker points out that one does not necessarily have to write about the event. Confessing it to someone else will have the same effect.

The rules for writing such confessions are simple:

1. Write for twenty minutes, for four consecutive days.

2. Write continuously about the most upsetting experience or trauma of your entire life.

3. Don't worry about grammar, spelling, or structure of the piece.

4. Write your deepest thoughts and emotions regarding the experience. Include all the details you remember and insights into the events.

Marriage As an Immune System Booster

Researchers Janice Kiecolt-Glaser and Ronald Glaser have conducted several studies that point to the immunological benefits of a happy marriage. In one study, the researchers compared the immune responses among married women who were evaluated for the quality of their relationships with their husbands. The same study also compared these married women to women who had been recently separated or divorced. Within the married group, those with high-quality relationships had better immune responses to antigens than those with low-quality relationships. In general, the married women had higher overall immune responses and, specifically, natural killer cell responses than those who were separated or divorced. The married women also had a greater percentage of CD4 cells and a lower concentration of antibody to Epstein-Barr virus, a sign that the virus was held in check and was not able to flare up.

Within the separated or divorced group, those with a high level of attachment to the estranged spouse had poorer immune response to an antigen and a lower percentage of CD4 cells than those with a low level of attachment. The conclusions are clear: people who have undergone the trauma of divorce must find a way to express and come to terms with their inner pain, either through counseling, ongoing support from a special group, or friends, lest they risk immune system depression and physical illness.

Men Are As Vulnerable As Women — Perhaps More So

Similar results were obtained in a study of men. There were no differences found in the level of CD4 cells, but again, separated men had higher amounts of Epstein-Barr virus antibodies than married men, and unhappily married men had higher levels of antibodies than those who were happily married. The separated men also were ill more often.

Among the men who were recently separated, those who initiated the separation had a better immune system profile and reported better health than the noninitiators did. The study was well controlled. Nutrition, weight, and sleep data did not differ between the married and separated groups; those who reported drug or alcohol abuse were excluded from the study. Therefore, such factors did not play a role in the study's results.

Men are particularly vulnerable to illness when they live alone or lose a loved one. Dr. Maradee Davis and her colleagues at the

INTIMACY AND RELATIONSHIPS

INTIMACY AND RELATIONSHIPS **163**

University of California at San Francisco studied 7,651 adults and found that middle-aged men who were unmarried or divorced were twice as likely to die within ten years than men who were married and lived with their wives. That finding held true even after accounting for differences in economic status, smoking habits, drinking habits, obesity, and physical activity.

"Men who lived alone or with someone other than a spouse had significantly shorter survival times compared with those living with a spouse," Dr. Davis reported in her study, published in the *American Journal of Public Health* (March 1992). The pattern of early death was particularly strong among younger men. "The age-adjusted relative hazard of dying was highest in the youngest age group, forty-five to fifty-four years, and decreased somewhat with increasing age."

This research points to the special vulnerability we all face when we are separated from someone we were deeply attached to or still love. It also reveals the unique psychological and physical risks to health that being alone can pose. As we said at the outset of this chapter, humans naturally seek intimacy, both with themselves and with another. Such intimacy supports good health. The loss of it takes both a psychological toll and a physical one.

The best recommendation, therefore, is this: if you have recently broken off a long-standing relationship, especially a marriage, do not isolate yourself from friends or loved ones. After such a trauma, people tend to wall themselves off from those who care about them. We might feel shamed by the events and feel we must assure people that we can make it on our own. All too often, our unhealthy message to the world is this: "I don't need help. I'm not that wounded and I can recover on my own." Very often, we are wounded far more than we let on, even to ourselves. We must take such pain seriously if we are to recover as quickly and efficiently as possible. Therefore, it is wise to seek out counseling and friends, to accept social invitations and the extended hand of those who love us.

A Sense of Community

We yearn not only for intimacy, but also for a sense of having a place in the world. In short, virtually all of us want and need community. Studies show that people who enjoy a strong sense of such support have enhanced lymphocyte activity, lower levels of antibodies to herpes virus, and greater natural killer cell activity. Overall, studies have shown that both cellular and humoral immunity are stronger when a person feels connected to community; conversely, people who feel isolated and alone have higher rates of cancer and infections.

One of the earliest and most impressive studies to demonstrate the need for social support and a sense of community was the Alameda County Study, which followed seven thousand residents of Alameda County, California, over a nine-year period. The study showed a direct relationship between social ties and longevity. Those who were married or had close personal friends or who sustained church or civic affiliations were more likely to live longer than those who were unmarried or socially isolated.

Numerous studies have shown that people who feel isolated have three to five times the mortality rate (not only from cardiovascular diseases, but from all causes) in comparison to people who don't feel isolated. Interestingly, this mortality rate is usually independent of blood cholesterol level, blood pressure, and even whether or not a person smokes.

Cancer and Social Support

A well-known, widely reported study of the healing effects of a support group was carried out by Stanford psychiatrist Dr. David

Spiegel and his colleague James L. Spira, Ph.D. In 1989, Spiegel reported that women with advanced breast cancer who participated in a support group lived twice as long as those who did not participate in such a group. Spiegel stresses the need for people to feel safe in the group. Initially, many worry that if they say what they truly believe, they will hurt someone else in the group — which might affect the progress of their disease — or they may be emotionally or psychologically injured themselves. Such concerns are remedied by the strong, active role taken by Spiegel and Spira, who guide discussions in such a way that everyone can share feelings without excessive worry.

In general, health-related groups have proved valuable, especially in improving the quality of life, enhancing coping skills, and reducing anxiety and depression. They serve as a support, comfort, and information source for people who share a common illness, such as cancer or AIDS. They also provide a setting in which to discuss the emotional impact of the illness, its meaning, various family difficulties caused by the disease (such as problems of intimacy), and the sense of isolation and stigma that frequently accompanies major illness. In general, support groups have been shown to result in fewer visits to doctors and hospitals by group participants.

Sandra Levy and her colleagues have followed a group of women with early breast cancer for seven years and found that social support predicted higher natural killer cell activity and the rate at which the disease progressed after recurrence. The level of active natural killer cells in the bloodstream was highly predictive of how quickly or slowly the disease would recur, or whether it would recur at all. Those with high levels of natural killer cells — which are central to the body's efforts to fight cancer — were found either to postpone the recurrence of the disease or to avoid recurrence entirely.

Social Support and Stress from Illness

Few things isolate people as much as disease. Whether you are taking care of someone who is ill or suffering from an illness yourself, the level of stress can be enormous. For people caring for patients with Alzheimer's disease, many of whom were spouses, immune system function tended to decline over time; however, it did so less in those with better social support networks and also in those who were not as distressed by the dementia-related behaviors. The spouses of cancer patients with good social support had better natural killer cell activity and better overall lymphocyte responsiveness than those with less adequate social support. Finally, breast cancer patients themselves had better natural killer cell activity if their perceived level of social support from spouse, physician, or friends was higher. Natural killer cell activity was also higher in those who used social support as a coping strategy.

Bereavement and the Immune System

We call it "dying of a broken heart," and indeed the research consistently shows that the loss of a loved one is associated with a depressed immune response and premature death. Studies have shown that bereavement specifically reduces the effectiveness of lymphocytes, a type of white blood cell essential to immune function. In some cases, the lymphocytes proliferate in a feeble way when stimulated. The net effect is that the person is incapable of warding off an illness that, for many, results in death.

One of the pioneering studies in the field of psychoneuroimmunology reported that lymphocytes from bereaved spouses had a reduced ability to proliferate in the face of a mitogen, possibly predisposing the bereaved person to illness. It was thought that this might contribute to the increased rate of illness in men who have lost their mates.

More recently, a number of studies have concentrated not so much on mood, but rather more directly on the importance of social support and relationships. The findings consistently show that intimate relationship or a broader social network protects the immune system, whereas discord in a personal relationship has the opposite effect. Social support protects the immune system, both during times of stress, such as a family illness, as well as under normal conditions.

"I am coming to believe that anything that promotes isolation leads to chronic stress and, in turn, may lead to illnesses like heart disease," says Dean Ornish, M.D., author of *Reversing Heart Disease* (1990). "Anything that promotes a sense of intimacy, community, and connection can be healing."

Intimacy Can Save Your Life

Ornish's words find resonance in a recent study done at Duke University Medical School. Redford Williams, M.D., director of behavioral research at Duke, found that those who suffer a heart attack and have no spouse or close personal friend are three times more likely to have a fatal heart attack within five years of the original event than those whose hearts are equally injured but are married or have intimate relationships.

The Duke University research is based on a nine-year follow-up study of 1,368 patients who were initially admitted to Duke for cardiac catheterization to diagnose heart disease. For people with both minor and severe heart muscle damage following a heart attack, the results were consistent. Such people generally face about a 40 percent chance of dying within five years. But Dr. Williams found that those who were married or had a close intimate relationship reduced their risk of suffering a fatal heart attack to 20 percent, whereas those who lacked intimacy raised their chances of dying to 60 percent.

Research consistently shows that both women and men with poor social support are more likely to die than those with more social support. The relative degree of social support a sick person experiences is one of the factors that can predict the outcome of the illness. This is true of all serious illnesses, including cancer, ischemic heart disease, and stroke.

The research is particularly interesting in regard to women with breast cancer. Researchers wanted to know whether the longevity of survival depended not so much on social support, but on the stage at which the person was diagnosed. They found that women who live alone tend to be diagnosed at an earlier stage of the cancer than those living with someone else. Yet those who live alone most often die sooner. In other words, early diagnosis was not a factor in determining longevity.

At this point, no one knows *why* those who live with someone actually live longer, except that the finding supports the general conclusion that those who have intimacy and strong social support tend to have stronger immune responses.

Recommendations for Building Supportive Relationships

The research points directly to some clear social recommendations for improved immune system function. These are especially important if you are battling a disease and want to boost your immune system by developing a stronger social support network. Here are some suggestions for improving your immune response by nurturing yourself socially:

- Join a support group that meets a particular need. The Yellow Pages of every telephone book contain a section called Social and Human Services that offers a wide variety of social support groups and services, including the American Friends Service Committee, family and child services, groups for people with AIDS, twelve-step programs such as Alcoholics Anonymous, Adult Children of Alcoholics (Al-Anon), and Overeaters Anonymous; programs and support for disabled people; groups that address coping with illnesses such as breast cancer and AIDS; groups for the elderly; gay, lesbian, and bisexual support groups; men's support groups; women's support groups; and helping organizations such as the United Way. The opening pages of the telephone book also include a self-help guide to support services offered in your community.

- Call local social clubs and organizations, such as the YMCA, the YWCA, B'nai B'rith, Hillel, and other social and religious organizations, to learn about programs and groups that fit your needs.

- Seek out personal professional counseling.

- Put an ad in the personals column in your local newspaper. Be specific about who you are and the kind of person or persons you are looking for.

- Answer an ad in the personals column of your local newspaper.

- Go dancing at the local swing, country, square, contra, circle, or African dance programs. See your local newspaper for listings.

- Become part of your religious community, and participate in the clubs, classes, and groups within that community.

- Talk to your doctor, minister, priest, or rabbi about ongoing support groups that will meet your particular desires or needs.

- Form your own men's or women's group. Find members by placing an ad in your local newspaper.

- Join a local choir.

- Join a writers' or poets' workshop, and write about what is occurring in your life. Writers' workshops are open to writers of all calibers and experience. Many are designed for people dealing with illness who wish to write about their experiences. See your local daily or weekly newspaper for listings.
- Volunteer at your local hospital.
- Surf the Internet.
- Become active in a cause you believe in, such as the arts, the environment, men's or women's issues, or health or political issues.
- Take a class at your local community college or at an adult education program. Catalogues are usually offered free to anyone who inquires by telephone.
- Take an aerobic exercise, swimming, or tennis class.
- Get to know your neighbor.

CHAPTER TWELVE

Immune System Booster #9: Staying Out of Harm's Way

D RUG, ALCOHOL, AND TOBACCO use are all associated with immunity-related illnesses, and, as the research demonstrates, there's little wonder. People who use drugs, abuse alcohol, and smoke are essentially cutting the legs out from under their immune systems. Consequently, when they encounter a virus, bacterium, or a form of cancer, they lack the resistance to ward it off.

In addition to the known toxins that we encounter each day, many substances that we judge to be harmless and even acceptable are, in fact, wolves in sheep's clothing. Not only do they depress immune response, but also they can contribute directly to disease. We all need to know about such substances if we are to protect ourselves against their deleterious side effects.

This chapter could just as well have been titled "Conscious Living," because its intention is to alert you to many of the avoidable poisons in your world. By staying away from these toxins, you can lighten the load on your body's defenses and thereby allow your immune system to direct its incredible powers more efficiently against any disease that your body may have to deal with. Understanding the effects of these and other substances is the basis for conscious living, which in turn is the foundation for health and longevity in the modern world.

Alcohol and the Immune System

More than an average of three alcoholic drinks per day is associated with an increased risk of stroke, high blood pressure, and several types of cancer, including cancer of the mouth, esophagus, liver, and breast. Light liquors, such as vodka, are as likely as dark liquors to lead to cancer.

Surprisingly, drinking some alcohol is associated with better health and longevity than not drinking at all. People who drink one to two drinks per day live longer than teetotalers. No one knows why entirely, except that alcohol increases HDL (the good cholesterol) and lowers the rate of coronary heart disease. The important guideline for alcohol consumption is moderation.

Many point to the well-known "French paradox" as proof that copious alcohol consumption allows people to consume high levels of fat. But this idea is simply fantasy and wishful thinking. The argument goes like this: in spite of high levels of animal fat in their diet, the French have a low level of heart disease because, it is argued, they drink lots of wine. According to this rationale, the wine somehow balances the fat.

In fact, the French who eat a great deal of animal fat also have high rates of heart disease. Also, the research shows that the French had lower rates of heart disease when their diets were based largely on grains, vegetables, fruit, and wine, with only small amounts of animal foods. Since the 1950s, however, the fat content of the French diet has steadily increased, as has the rate of heart disease and other degenerative illnesses. Older French people do indeed experience lower rates of heart disease, but their diet was considerably lower in fat than that of the younger generation of today. The modern French, unfortunately, will debunk their own myth — the French paradox will run out on them within the next twenty years.

This is not to say that wine contains no health-promoting ingredients. Like green and black tea, wine contains antioxidants and bioflavonoids that protect the body from both heart disease and cancer. These substances may make blood platelets less sticky, which prevents the formation of cholesterol plaques and blood clots, or microthrombi, which cause most heart attacks. Red wine contains more antioxidants and bioflavonoids than white. Although wine does have some positive immune and cardiovascular effects, they are overridden when the diet is high in fat. The best advice, therefore, is to drink moderate amounts of alcohol (if you drink at all) and keep the fat content of your diet low.

One drink does not appear to suppress immunity, but three or more do; immune system suppression increases as the quantity of alcohol consumed increases. Some people, such as those with asthma, appear to be particularly sensitive to the effects of alcohol. Lymphocytes, macrophages, and granulocytes are all affected by high doses of alcohol, leaving heavy alcohol users less able to fight infections.

In nonalcoholics, the effects of alcohol seem to be short-lived, and the immune system returns to normal within a day, as alcohol is cleared from the body. However, before the alcohol is fully eliminated, it can have a damaging effect on the immune system. People with alcohol in their bloodstreams who are in accidents, for example, are more likely to develop infections and other complications. Since drinking and accidents seem to go together, this scenario actually is quite common and makes recovery more difficult.

Because of their impaired immunity, alcoholics are much more susceptible to infections. Immune system depression occurs in alcoholics before liver disease develops, and is compounded because they tend to suffer from nutritional deficiencies, including low levels of zinc, beta-carotene, and other carotenoids. Poor nutrition and smoking add to the effects of alcohol on immunity.

When alcoholics quit drinking, their immune defects are at least partly reversed over a period of months.

Alcohol, Pregnancy, and Immune System Depression

Women who drink large amounts of alcohol during pregnancy run the risk of causing fetal alcohol syndrome in an unborn child. Children born with this disease have low immune responses and are at greater risk of infection throughout childhood. Scientists believe that the effects of prenatal alcohol on the immune system are secondary to the hormonal changes caused by the alcohol during development. These hormonal changes in turn depress immunity and predispose the children to disease. More than two drinks per day increases levels of cortisol, a hormone that dulls immune responses in the mother. This and other hormonal changes alter the development of the neuroendocrine system in the fetus. Infants with fetal alcohol syndrome are born with distorted faces and often suffer from learning disabilities as well.

Breast-feeding usually helps transfer protective immunity from a mother to her infant. Much of this effectiveness is lost, however, if the mother continues to drink heavily when she is nursing.

Psychoactive Recreational Drugs and the Immune System

Cocaine

Both human and animal studies show that cocaine suppresses immunity. People who use cocaine have fewer circulating CD4 cells, yet, surprisingly, more natural killer cells for several days after cocaine use. The ability of granulocytes to move toward a chemical signal sent out by CD4 cells and macrophages is also decreased, suggesting that the immune system is uncoordinated and lacks responsiveness.

In animal studies, cocaine has been shown to suppress the ability of macrophages and CD4 cells to kill pathogens and cancer cells and to weaken the capacity of these cells to produce cytokines. It takes several days for the immunity-depressing effects of cocaine to wear off, and the higher the dose of cocaine used, the longer it takes for the immune system to recover. The disruption caused by cocaine makes the user susceptible to infections and cancer.

Cocaine and alcohol are especially harmful when used together. The two combine to create a compound called cocaethylene, which suppresses lymphocyte function more than either cocaine or alcohol when used alone.

Heroin, Morphine, and Methadone

Intravenous (IV) drug users manifest several different kinds of immune system abnormalities. Their lymphocytes respond less effectively to a challenge, their CD4 counts are lower than those of nonusers, and they have higher antibodies to viruses and other antigens.

Pregnancy and IV Drug Use

Like alcohol use, IV drug use can weaken the immune systems of the babies of women who use drugs during pregnancy. The infants have fewer CD4 cells in ratio to CD8 cells (the suppressor cells), and their immunity profiles resemble those of their drug-addicted mothers.

Marijuana

Marijuana suppresses the immune system when used chronically. However, when used occasionally, it is the least immunosuppressive of the mood-altering drugs. Most studies of marijuana have examined the effect of its major psychoactive component, delta-tetrahydrocannabinol (DTHC). In animal studies, repeated exposure to DTHC over a period of weeks suppresses the effectiveness of natural killer cells and interferon production, which weakens the body's fight against bacterial infection and cancer. However, a single exposure to DTHC has no measurable effect on immunity.

Heavy use of marijuana may lead to a greater susceptibility to infections and cancer.

Other Psychoactive Recreational Drugs

Other recreational drugs are less well studied, but scattered reports suggest that LSD, PCP, amphetamines, and nitrite inhalants ("poppers") can all be immunosuppressive.

Nitrite inhalants have lowered the number of T cells in human blood and inhibited natural killer cell activity. In animal studies, exposure reduced the ability to produce antibodies. It also reduced the ability of macrophages to kill cancer cells and tumors. This might be one reason that nitrite inhalants have been associated with the development of the cancer Kaposi's sarcoma in HIV-infected men.

■ ■ ■

Virtually all recreational drugs suppress immunity if used frequently enough; the least impact occurs when the drug was used only once or twice per month.

Medications are available to help a person stop using drugs. Acupuncture has been shown to relieve symptoms of withdrawal from heroin and cocaine use, even for people who had been severe abusers.

Tobacco and the Immune System

Smoking is associated with a number of major diseases including cancer and heart disease. It is estimated that at least one in seven cases of cancer is caused by smoking: one in four for men, one in twenty-five for women. In 1987, lung cancer became the leading cause of death in women, following the increase in women smokers in the 1950s. Each cigarette smoked is said to cost $5\frac{1}{2}$ minutes of life. Fortunately, people who stop smoking diminish their risk of contracting all smoking-related illnesses.

Passive smoke increases disease in those who share space with smokers. Sadly, children whose mothers smoke suffer twice as many respiratory infections during their first year than children whose mothers do not smoke. Smoking by mothers or fathers also increases the risk of sudden infant death syndrome by two to three times the average rate.

The effects of smoking are cumulative. The more you smoke and the longer you smoke, the weaker your immune system becomes.

Macrophages from the lungs of smokers are unable to protect them against disease. They are far less capable of destroying viruses, bacteria, and cancer cells, and their ability to produce cytokines and communicate with CD4 cells is drastically diminished. The ability of granulocytes to phagocytize is also weakened. These conditions make smokers susceptible to cancer and respiratory infections.

Not surprisingly, the combination of nicotine and alcohol is more suppressive to the immune system than either one alone.

Tobacco stimulates production of antibodies that trigger inflammation and allergic reactions, which is probably why smokers experience more allergies than nonsmokers. Other effects of smoking include a decrease in blood levels of vitamin C and beta-carotene.

Smoking Cessation and Immune Response

Fortunately, the immune system begins to return to normal within a few months after smoking stops, even in people who have smoked for years. Withdrawal symptoms last for one to two weeks. The first three days are the hardest. Nicotine patches or inhaling black pepper oil reduces the craving in some people.

Pharmaceutical Medications and the Immune System

Prescription drugs and over-the-counter medications are generally helpful when taken as directed, but they often have side effects. Relatively few medications have been studied to determine their effect on the immune system. Several classes of drugs, however, are immunosuppressive. Foremost among these are glucocorticoids such as cortisol and dexamethasone, both used for treating asthma and allergic reactions. These are so immunosuppressive that they have been used to suppress the immune systems of people who undergo transplant operations and of people with inflammatory diseases. They leave users highly susceptible to infections.

Antibiotics

Some antibiotics suppress immunity, whereas others stimulate it. In many cases, antibiotics replace immune system function by shutting down certain immune responses. For example, clindamycin, roxithromycin, and trimethoprim, all common antibiotics, prevent granulocytes from producing chemicals that kill most bacteria. Mezlocillin, rifampicin, prodigiosin, and doxycycline inhibit T lymphocyte functions.

Long-term use of these and other common antibiotics can result in weakened immune system function. Moreover, antibiotics also kill friendly intestinal flora, bacteria the body depends on to help break down and digest food. When these bacteria are killed, they are often replaced by harmful *Candida albicans* and parasitic bacteria that contribute to disease. *Candida albicans,* of course, gives rise to yeast infections, or candidiasis. These organisms thrive in immunity-depressed environments and consequently cause much suffering in people with HIV infection.

At least one antibiotic, ciprofloxacin, stimulates production of cytokines, which promotes the immune response.

Anesthetics

A number of drugs used as anesthetics are immunosuppressive, among them thiopental, halothane, Avertin, isoflurane, and ketamine. Their use may contribute to the well-known immunosuppressive effects of surgery, which leave patients more vulnerable to infections.

Penicillin and Autoimmune Disease

Penicillin and sulfa drugs can trigger autoimmune diseases, which can be fatal. Such drugs bring on illnesses by attaching themselves to the surface of red blood cells, causing the cells to appear foreign to the immune system and thus stimulating an immune response against one's own blood. One of the illnesses that can be caused by penicillin is hemolytic anemia, a potentially lethal disease. Usually red cells recover once penicillin is stopped, and new red cells, which do not carry penicillin on their surfaces, replace the old.

Environmental Toxins and the Immune System

The study of environmental toxins constitutes a relatively new area of research; the majority of papers have appeared in the past three to four years. Among the most widely studied compounds are herbicides, such as dioxin and benzopyrene; those found in automobile exhaust; and the chemicals that make up the smoke from industrial and municipal plants. All of these can depress CD4 cell and macrophage activities and can interfere with the production of both B cells and T cells.

Other pollutants shown to be immunosuppressive are ozone and sulfuric acid, found in acid rain. Both chemicals impair the function of macrophages in the lungs, leaving us more susceptible to respiratory infections. Both decrease the ability of immune cells to gobble up pathogens and cancer cells, and they prevent optimal production of tumor necrosis factor.

Heavy Metals

Certain heavy metals also suppress the immune response. In animal models, aluminum and mercury both impair the ability of T lymphocytes to produce cytokines. Both have been shown to induce autoimmune disease in laboratory animals.

Ultraviolet Light

Ultraviolet rays induce mutations and prevent CD4 cells from recognizing and destroying tumor cells.

Conversely, people with psoriasis and other related skin conditions benefit from ultraviolet light, in part because it inhibits the immune system's inflammatory reactions that cause the affliction.

■ ■ ■

Most drugs and toxins can be avoided, or exposure to them can be minimized. We can drink moderate amounts of alcohol or avoid it entirely. When faced with a situation in which exposure to polluted air is unavoidable, we can increase antioxidants and other immunity-boosting nutrients and foods described in previous chapters. Whenever possible, get out into the fresh air and walk; it allows the body to eliminate some of the accumulated waste from the lungs.

The best rule of thumb is to recognize the dangers in our world and avoid them whenever you can. If you can't avoid them, compensate by boosting your immune system.

CHAPTER THIRTEEN

Immune System Booster #10: Creating Balance

I F YOU THINK THAT balance in life is important and truly value the time you spend playing and relaxing as much as the time you spend working and being productive, you will live in virtual opposition to the ethics of modern life. Most of us are driven to produce, always running out of time and deprived of sleep. We compensate ourselves with material rewards and an inner belief that we are better people for our productivity, our accomplishments, and our work ethic. Yet despite the social reinforcement that this behavior receives, we still hear, if only fleetingly, that small voice within that encourages us to spend more time playing, or praying, or listening to music, or being with loved ones, or simply getting more sleep. Our response to that voice, all too often, is to demean such activities as unimportant or unnecessary — or even a waste of time.

The study of the immune system is teaching us that balance is essential to good health. We are learning the lesson from many different angles, from the purely physical, to the psychological, and even to the spiritual. We have already seen, for example, that certain nutrients and behaviors that boost the immune system, when taken to excess, actually depress immune response. Zinc, for example, is essential to a healthy immune response when consumed in doses of about fifteen milligrams. But when consumption exceeds that amount, the nutrient weakens immunity.

In the case of people infected with HIV, excesses of vitamin A speed the progress of the disease to full-blown AIDS. Yet when consumed in moderation, vitamin A is essential to a healthy immune system, especially for people with HIV. Moderate exercise boosts immunity, but excesses depress immune response. Even alcohol is harmless — and perhaps health enhancing — when consumed in moderation — but it is clearly destructive in excess. Too much of a good thing is not such a good thing.

Balance is a way of being that can be applied to every aspect of our lives. It is a guide to how you do ordinary things: whether you stroll or power-walk; whether you play to win or play for the fun and the workout; whether or not you can alternate your styles — playing to win sometimes, and just playing for fun at others.

Balance determines how we experience time and even whether we feel that we have enough time. One of the paradoxes of modern life is that the more we hurry, the more under stress we are and the less time we seem to have. Balance determines the quality of our relationships. It teaches us to listen, as well as to speak, to be passive as well as aggressive, to give as well as to receive.

Ultimately, balance is about trust and even faith. Somehow it encourages a positive attitude toward others and ourselves. People intuitively know that a person with a balanced view of situations tends to be just.

An *imbalanced* view of life is focused mostly on the negative consequences of situations and events. The more imbalanced our perspective, the more we worry about how things can go wrong and how such mishaps will affect our lives. The more imbalanced our lives, the more we are pressed to focus on issues of survival — we are duped into believing we must control ourselves and others to an unreasonable degree. We cannot foster intimacy with ourselves and with others. An imbalanced life is ultimately driven by fear.

Be Good to Your Body

Balance is also a key to how you take care of your body. Do you demand more of your body than you are willing to give in return? Practices such as yoga, tai chi chuan, stretching, and massage are gentle ways of giving back to the body, ways of nourishing it with physical caring. These practices relieve the body of tension and the effects of stress. Despite the fact that there is little hard scientific evidence for the positive effects of such practices, we know intuitively that they provide us with a kind of physical, psychological, and spiritual nourishment that raises the quality of our lives and even affects our health.

This is why people who become sick invariably try to reestablish balance in their lives in order to recover their health. People who have been driven in their careers and suddenly experience a health crisis turn to home and family and the simple pleasures of life as a way of recovery. Type A people, for example, often recognize their extreme behaviors and attitudes as a cause of their disease. In response, they return to a simpler existence that is ultimately more satisfying.

Without balance, none of the immune system boosters we've discussed can be used effectively. We might get too much of a single nutrient and exercise too vigorously for good health. We might neglect loved ones and friends. In the end, balance is the key to this program.

Seek Out Small Pleasures

Stress narrows your focus. It can make you lose perspective, causing the stressful situation to eclipse the rest of your life. This dynamic can have a strong impact on immunity. On the other hand, taking time out to enjoy a pleasant event — going out with friends, enjoying a favorite meal, seeing a humorous movie —

can boost your immune response for as long as two days, according to research conducted by scientists at the State University of New York (SUNY) Medical School. For three months, researchers followed one hundred men who encountered numerous stressful events, such as being criticized at work by the boss, which depressed these men's immune response. Other stressful situations included conflicts with fellow employees, pressures of overwork and deadlines, and frustrating chores at home. The SUNY researchers found that immune function was depressed for approximately twenty-four hours after each stressful encounter.

However, events such as family celebrations, having friends over for dinner, fishing, or jogging all boosted immune response for two days. "Positive events seem to have a stronger helpful impact on immune function than upsetting events do a negative one," said Dr. Arthur Stone, a psychologist at SUNY who conducted the research. Stone and his colleagues found that whenever the men reported having a cold, there was a parallel increase in the number of undesirable events from three to five days before the cold symptoms manifested themselves. At the same time, there was a drop in the desirable events on those days.

Get a Good Night's Sleep

One of the big problems with being driven by time is that many of us are deprived of adequate sleep, which depresses the immune system. One of the first steps in achieving balance is getting enough sleep.

The immune system has a normal circadian rhythm in which the number of immune cells in the blood rise and fall throughout the day. Other changes also take place throughout the day, such as cytokine production, the ability of cells to proliferate, and hormone levels. For instance, cortisol levels are highest in the morning and fall throughout the day. Interestingly, in studies in which sequential blood samples were taken over a twenty-four-hour period, the circadian pattern revealed changes in immune system function to suggest increases and decreases in immune cells. At certain times during the day, immune function may be lower than normal, but at other times it may be normal or higher than normal.

One of the major rhythms of the body, of course, is the sleep cycle. Although no one understands how sleep works, it seems to be a time when the mind and body can restore themselves in the absence of daily demands that distract them. During sleep, interleukin-1 levels rise, which is consistent with the purpose of this cytokine, since it induces sleep whenever we are ill.

Several studies in which participants were kept awake for forty-eight hours or longer show that sleep deprivation disturbs the immune system. The effects of sleep deprivation differ among the various studies, but in general, immunity is depressed. Specifically, lymphocyte proliferation, phagocytosis, cytokine production, and natural killer cell activity were found to be lower than normal.

Few studies have explored the role of sleep on immune function under normal circumstances. One such study by Michael Irwin and colleagues showed that normal variations in sleep may also have relevance to immunity. Irwin studied depressed and normal people in a sleep laboratory. There, he measured not only total sleep time, but also sleep efficiency and various stages of sleep, including total non-REM sleep. He found that for both controls and depressed subjects, natural killer cell activity was positively correlated with total, as well as non-REM, sleep. He concluded that in order to maintain good natural killer cell activity, we all need a good night's sleep to help fight off viral infections and prevent the development or spread of cancer.

Research confirms that the aroma of oil of lavender helps people get to sleep, so if you are having difficulty nodding off, you might try placing a lavender sachet on your pillow. A program of frequent exercise can also help regularize sleeping patterns. Melatonin can also help you get to sleep; 0.1–0.3 milligrams will be enough if only a little help is needed, but insomniacs may need 2–6 milligrams. Melatonin also boosts the immune system by counteracting the effects of stress.

■ ■ ■

Balance is truly the key to success in boosting your immune system. The next chapter provides a flexible program that brings together all the immune system boosters to help you maintain and improve your health.

CHAPTER FOURTEEN

A Program for Boosting the Immune System

E ACH CHAPTER OF THIS BOOK contains recommendations regarding a specific nutrient or behavior. In this chapter, we put those recommendations together for you and offer a
week's menu of ideas on how immunity-boosting practices can
be woven into your life. Like any other set of habits, a healthy
lifestyle becomes second nature with a little time and consistent
effort. Give yourself that time. Allow yourself the flexibility and
the latitude to learn to prepare these foods and grow accustomed
to their tastes; to incorporate certain behaviors, such as meditation and exercise, into your daily life; and to seek out the kinds of
social support you need.

All change is scary. It helps to keep a journal. Write down the
areas of your life you'd like to improve; also record the fears you
have that surround such changes. Each day, spend a few minutes
recording your progress and your setbacks. In time, you will become so intimate with yourself that such writing will be very
much like writing about a friend, one for whom you have tremendous compassion and admiration. As we discussed in Chapter
10, writing resolves inner conflicts and integrates long-repressed
parts of us. It brings the inner peace and centeredness that can
come only with self-knowledge. At the same time, writing will
also help you adapt to the program we've provided.

You do not have to adopt the entire program all at once. Nor must you adopt it in its entirety to benefit from it. Lots of choices are offered. Start with the practices you are most comfortable with. Some people find it easier to make changes one step at a time; for others a total switch all at once is the better approach. The more you incorporate these recommendations into your life, the greater the benefits you will accrue.

Rather than reiterate what has already been said in each chapter, we have tried to create a diet, exercise, and mind-body program that streamlines these ideas into an accessible, practical plan of action. The diet, for example, contains the antioxidants, minerals, herbs, and cancer-fighting foods we have already discussed. Lifestyle suggestions include time for meditation and exercise.

A Summary of Recommended Immune System Boosters

The following is a summary of recommended immune system boosters. For more ways to incorporate them into your life, especially immunity-boosting and cancer-fighting foods, see the cooking instructions and menu plans that follow.

Immune System Booster #1

Eat plenty of foods rich in the following antioxidants:

- Foods containing beta-carotene, including dark green, yellow, and orange vegetables. Eat at least two servings of one or more of these vegetables daily.
- Vegetables and fruits that contain vitamin C, such as broccoli, green pepper, cabbage, collard greens, and citrus fruits. Eat at least one serving of these daily.
- Grains and vegetables containing vitamin E, especially seeds

and nuts, whole wheat bread, brown rice, sweet potatoes, and beans. Eat at least two servings of them daily.

Immune System Booster #2

To get adequate minerals, make the following foods a staple part of your daily and weekly diet:

- Whole grains, such as whole wheat, brown rice, barley, corn, millet, oats, and buckwheat. Eat two servings of a whole grain food daily.
- Green vegetables.
- Beans, tofu, tempeh, and other bean products.
- Fish and shellfish.
- Seeds and nuts.
- Sea vegetables (seaweed). Include small amounts (one to two tablespoons) at least three times per week.

Immune System Booster #3

Eat a diet low in fat.

- Choose fish and chicken instead of red meat; if you do eat red meat, do so no more than once per week, and keep the portions small, about three ounces (the size of a deck of cards).
- Make the majority of your diet vegetable foods, especially whole grains, fresh vegetables, beans, and whole grain snacks.
- Eat a high-fiber diet. Fiber binds with fat in the intestinal tract and causes it to be eliminated from the body.

Immune System Booster #4

Include immunity-boosting herbs and condiments in your diet, especially the following ones:

- Eat two to three shiitake or reishi mushrooms two or three times per week. Some people find that eating more than eight per week causes stomach upsets.
- Eat cooked or raw garlic three to five times per week.
- Drink at least one cup daily of black or green tea.
- Include at least one serving of cruciferous vegetables per day.
- Serve soybeans, tofu, tempeh, or other soybean products four times per week.
- Eat beans five times per week (this can include various soybean products).
- Use the other recommended herbs and spices especially when your immune system needs boosting, such as when you feel affected by a cold, the flu, or some other illness.

Immune System Booster #5

Exercise at least four times per week.

- Walk at least four times per week.
- Enjoy some other aerobic activity regularly, such as a competitive sport, bicycling, dancing, and so on.

Immune System Booster #6

Practice stress reduction techniques. Choose one that appeals to you and gives you a sense of internal calm and peace. Among the most powerful stress reduction activities are the following:

- Meditation
- Prayer
- Progressive relaxation exercises
- Diaphragmatic breathing
- Positive imaging and affirmation
- Long-distance running

Immune System Booster #7

Develop positive attitudes toward other people and toward life in general.

- Write in a journal or diary daily.
- Confess traumas and painful memories to your journal or to someone you trust and can confide in, such as a long-standing friend, counselor, priest, minister, or rabbi.
- Learn to deal effectively with anger. (See recommendations in Chapter 10.)
- Seek out a healer.

Immune System Booster #8

Seek out supportive groups and social outlets.

- Join a support group that focuses on issues of special concern to you.
- Join a social, ethnic, or religious club or organization.
- Become a member of a religious community in which you can find support.
- Become active in a cause you believe in.

Immune System Booster #9

As much as possible, avoid toxins in your environment.

- Do not smoke cigarettes.
- Avoid all recreational drugs.
- Avoid all needless over-the-counter and prescription medication.
- Avoid or minimize exposure to toxic environments.

Immune System Booster #10

Practice balance in everyday life.

- If you take vitamin and mineral supplements, take only small amounts that meet the recommended daily allowance for that particular nutrient, with the possible exception of vitamin E.
- Drink alcohol moderately (no more than one or two drinks daily, if you drink at all).
- Find the small pleasures in life, and revel in them.
- Get adequate sleep.

■ ■ ■

Let's turn now to the specifics of a lifestyle that boosts the immune system, beginning with a healthy diet. Cooking instructions are offered throughout.

The Immunity-Boosting Diet

Whole Grains

Make whole grain the center of at least one meal per day. Whole grains are rich in vitamin E, complex carbohydrates (for long-lasting energy), fiber (for healthy digestion), and other essential nutrients.

Recommended Grains

- *Barley.* Both whole grain and "pearled" barley, which is lightly refined, are wonderful in soups and stews, or cooked with a variety of other hearty vegetables and beans, such as carrots, onions, leeks, and shiitake mushrooms. It is delicious when cooked in a miso or tamari-shoyu broth.

- *Brown rice.* You can choose short-, medium-, or long-grain rice. Brown rice is prepared by pressure cooking or boiling.
- *Buckwheat.* Forms of buckwheat include groats, noodles such as soba, and flour products such as pancake mixes. Buckwheat can be cooked with sauerkraut and a variety of vegetables, including carrots and onions.
- *Millet.* This grain can be boiled or pressure-cooked by itself, or cooked with a variety of vegetables, especially cauliflower, carrots, and other grains, such as barley or rice.
- *Oats.* Oats can be purchased whole, steel-cut, or rolled. Boiled as a breakfast cereal, oats can be combined with a variety of fruits or eaten plain.
- *Whole wheat.* The list of sources of whole wheat is seemingly endless: wheat berries, bulgur, *fu* (baked puffed-wheat gluten), *seitan* (kneaded wheat gluten, meaty and hearty), whole wheat bread, chapati (an Indian bread), and whole wheat pastas and noodles, including *udon.*

Ideas for Preparing Grains

Noodle Soup: First, bring a pot of water to boil. Add *udon* (a whole wheat noodle) or soba (buckwheat) noodles, shiitake mushrooms, and vegetables to the broth. Boil the contents for about twenty minutes, until the noodles are cooked. Turn off the flame, and add tamari, shoyu, or miso to the broth. This dish is rich in nutrition and a wonderful way to include shiitake mushrooms in your diet. A very immunity-boosting one-pot meal.

How to Pressure-Cook Brown Rice: For every two cups of brown rice, use three and a half to four cups of water; add a pinch of sea salt. Secure the lid on the pot, and turn on high flame. Bring it to pressure (which takes about ten minutes); once the regulator hisses intensely, turn the flame down to low, and cook the rice for forty to forty-five minutes. A stalk of *kombu* seaweed (very rich in minerals) can be used in place of sea salt. Rice also can be combined with other grains, such as millet or barley, or with beans, such as adzuki beans. Sweet brown rice is a glutinous form of brown rice that can be cooked with beans to make a rich, hearty dish.

Cooking Other Grains: Pressure cooking, boiling, steaming, frying, and baking are possible preparations. Use a pinch of sea salt when cooking grains to help them break down and make them easier to digest.

Vegetables

Vegetables are among the most abundant sources of minerals and vitamins on earth. A cup of cooked collard greens, for example, has more calcium than a cup of milk. Collard greens also provide carotenoids (including beta-carotene) and fiber, and they contain virtually no fat. Eat three to four vegetable dishes per day. The following list can help you make selections.

- Eat leafy green vegetables two times per day, especially those marked by an asterisk in the table on the next page.
- Eat at least one "round" or root vegetable daily, especially those marked by an asterisk in the table.
- Regularly eat vegetables rich in beta-carotene; these include squash, carrots, brussels sprouts, broccoli, and collard greens. All of these vegetables enhance immune response.
- Eat shiitake mushrooms regularly — two to four times per week — as a vegetable dish or in soup broths.

Vegetable Selections

Leafy Greens (twice per day)	Round Vegetables (once per day)	Root Vegetables (once per day)
asparagus	artichokes	burdock
beet greens	bamboo shoots	carrot*
carrot tops	beets	celery
chinese cabbage	broccoli*	chicory root
collard greens*	brussels sprouts*	daikon radish[1]
curly dock	cabbage*	dandelion root
dandelion greens	leeks	lotus root
endive	okra	onion
escarole	peas	parsnip*
kale*	shiitake mushrooms*	red radish
lamb's quarters[1]	snow peas	rutabaga*
leek greens	squashes*	turnip*
lettuce	butternut squash	
mustard greens*	hakkaido pumpkin[1]	
parsley	hubbard squash	
plantain[1]	pumpkin	
scallions	yellow squash	
shepherd's purse[1]	zucchini	
sorrel	string beans	
sprouts	sweet potatoes	
swiss chard	yams	
turnip greens		
watercress*		

---

1. Daikon radish is a large, long, mild form of radish used in Japanese cooking and good raw. Lamb's quarters, plantain, and shepherd's purse are wild leafy greens. Hakkaido pumpkin is a Japanese pumpkin similar to acorn squash.

Ideas for Preparing Vegetables

Steaming vegetables preserves nutrients, flavor, and texture. Most can be steamed for three to five minutes, depending on their size and consistency, in a half inch of water. You can also boil vegetables in water with a couple of drops of tamari or shoyu (optional) for three to five minutes. Nutrients are lost in greater quantities when vegetables are boiled in a larger volume of water over a longer period of time. Dense vegetables such as beets, however, do require longer cooking time. Reuse vegetable broth in soups and sauces to add nutrients.

You can sauté vegetables with good-quality oils (sesame is ideal). Lightly coat a frying pan, add washed and cut vegetables, and sauté for about five minutes.

Baking is the best way to prepare squashes. Cut up winter squash and then bake it at 375 to 400 degrees Fahrenheit for one to two hours until tender. Summer squash and zucchini require far less time — twenty to thirty-five minutes, depending on size. Bake yams and sweet potatoes at 400 to 500 degrees Fahrenheit for about one hour.

Beans (Legumes)

Beans are rich in protein, fiber, and phytoestrogens, which boost immunity and fight cancer. We recommend eating beans five times per week.

Consult a good recipe book for instructions for cooking beans. Many require soaking before they can be cooked. When you're in a hurry, you can open a can of precooked kidney beans or chickpeas, rinse them, and directly add them to a dish of grains or vegetables. Lentils cook quickly and do not require soaking. You can also add beans to your diet by incorporating soybean products into a variety of dishes. Consider tofu (firm or silken), *natto* (fermented soybean condiment), tempeh fried in sesame or olive oil, or miso as a flavoring for soup.

Experiment with a variety of beans; they vary in texture and flavor. Adzuki beans, black-eyed peas, chickpeas, kidney beans, lima beans, lentils (they come in different varieties), navy beans, pinto beans, soybeans, and split peas are a few suggestions; there are many others as well.

Ideas for Preparing Beans

- *Boiling.* This is the preferred method for cooking most beans. Soak dried beans (but don't soak lentils) overnight, and boil them with a single stalk of *kombu* seaweed, which will add minerals and cause the beans to be more digestible (it will not affect the flavor of the beans). Add a pinch of sea salt or a few drops of tamari or shoyu when the beans are 80 percent done. Boil for one and a half to two hours. You might add green peppers, onions, carrots, garlic, and basil for the last half hour of cooking. Make a large pot of beans, and reheat them for three or four meals.

- *Pressure cooking.* First, be sure that the pressure cooker regulator is clean. Beans can clog the regulator and cause problems in cooking. Add three cups of water per cup of beans; cook with a stalk of *kombu* seaweed. Cover the pressure cooker; lock it shut; bring it to pressure (indicated by the hissing of the regulator), which usually requires approximately ten minutes; reduce heat to low, and cook for forty-five minutes.

- *Baking.* Place beans in a pan of water, using three to four cups of water per cup of beans; add a stalk of *kombu* seaweed, if desired, and a pinch of sea salt. Bake at 350 degrees Fahrenheit for three to four hours. When beans are 80 percent done, add a variety of condiments or spices, such as raisins, tomato sauce, mustard, onions, miso, tamari, shoyu, or others.

Seaweeds

Sea vegetables are among the most abundant sources of minerals on earth. We recommend that you eat them three to five times per week. Eat only one- to two-tablespoon portions per serving. Rinse and soak seaweeds thoroughly before using them, to remove excess sodium. To adjust to the flavor of seaweed, try *sushi nori* seaweed. It does not require any preparation; simply remove it from package, wrap rice or other grains in the seaweed, and eat it like a sandwich. Later, you can try other seaweeds given in the following list, such as *wakame,* which is especially good in miso soup (a recipe follows this section). Seaweeds tend to taste of the ocean — salty and slightly fishy.

- *Alaria.* Cut this seaweed into small pieces, boil it for use in a particular dish, or add it to soups and stews; it should be cooked for thirty minutes. It is rich in vitamins B, C, and K, as well as many trace elements.
- *Arame.* Cook *arame* for thirty minutes with carrots, onions, and lemon juice, alone or in soups and stews. It supplies carbohydrates, calcium, and many other minerals.
- *Dulse.* This seaweed is rich in protein; vitamins A, C, E, and B; iodine; and iron and other trace minerals. *Dulse* can be roasted and added to rice and other grains as a condiment, or used as an ingredient in soups and stews.
- *Hijiki.* Loaded with nutrition, including protein, vitamins A and B, calcium, phosphorus, iron, and many trace minerals, *hijiki* can be boiled with carrots, onions, and daikon radishes for one to one and a half hours.

- *Irish moss.* Used as a thickening agent for soups and stews, it is rich in vitamins A and B₁, iron, sodium, calcium, and other trace elements.
- *Kombu.* Use a stalk when cooking beans to soften them and make the beans easier to digest. It can also be served as a vegetable with carrots, onions, rutabagas, turnips, and daikon radishes. *Kombu* is rich in many nutrients.
- *Nori.* This is perhaps the easiest sea vegetable to use and the one most acceptable to the novice palate. *Nori* comes in sheets and is used to make *nori* rolls, sushi, and rice balls (brown rice covered with *nori*). Roast *nori* over an open flame for five seconds; when it turns bright green, remove it from the flame. *Nori* also can be crumbled and used as a condiment. It supplies vitamins A, B, C, and D; calcium; phosphorus; iron; and trace elements.
- *Wakame.* This leafy, rich sea vegetable is used mostly in soups and stews. It cooks in twenty minutes and is very nutritious. It contains calcium, phosphorus, iron, potassium, and vitamins B and C.

Miso Soup

Eat miso soup up to five times per week. Miso is very rich in genistein, a cancer fighter. (See Chapter 7 for more on genistein and miso.) Experiment with a variety of misos. Though all include soybeans, they are fermented with different grains, such as rice and barley.

Recipe: Begin by adding a two-inch section of *wakame* seaweed for each cup of boiling water. Simmer. Cut vegetables (traditionally, carrots and onions are used, but you can add others) while the seaweed cooks, and then add the vegetables. Cook until the vegetables are soft — usually about twenty minutes. Reduce flame to low. Add approximately one-quarter to one-half teaspoon of miso per cup of broth, to taste; cook for a few minutes, and then serve hot.

Animal Foods

Throughout this book, the message is clear that decreasing intake of animal foods while increasing consumption of whole grains, vegetables, and fruits leads to boosted immune response and better health. Here are some recommendations for those who would like to lower, but not eliminate, their consumption of animal foods.

- Eat low-fat fish one to four times per week (or more, if desired). White fish is the most nutritious animal food. Cod, scrod, haddock, flounder, halibut, and sole are excellent choices. Occasionally serve shellfish, which is rich in minerals.

- Salmon is a healthful fish. White fish and salmon offer omega-3 polyunsaturated oils, which lower cholesterol level and may boost immunity, especially for HIV-positive people. (See Chapter 15 for more on fish oils and HIV.)

- Reduce or eliminate from your diet all red meat, dairy food, and eggs. All are rich in fat and cholesterol. If you choose to eliminate dairy food from a child's diet, be careful to ensure that the diet is adequate in the vitamins and minerals that dairy foods supply. Consult a nutritionist or your doctor.

- Minimize or eliminate poultry consumption. If you do eat poultry, eat organically grown chicken and turkey. The white meat is lower in fat than the dark. Avoid the skin, which is rich in fat.

Condiments and Dressings

Consider the following nutritious ways to add flavor to your foods. Your immune system will benefit. Except for oils and seeds, which should be used sparingly because of their fat content, these ingredients can be used in any amount, for a subtle or zingy effect.

- Garlic. (Use it raw, grated on vegetables, and also add it to your cooking.)
- Grated ginger root.
- Horseradish.
- Lemon juice, sliced lemons, lemon water.
- Miso-based dressings.
- Olive oil and tofu-based salad dressings.
- Rice vinegar.
- Sauerkraut.
- Scallions, chives, parsley.
- Seaweed shakes. (These are containers of seaweed flakes that can be purchased in natural foods stores and used instead of salt.)
- Sesame seeds. (Roast them in a dry frying pan while roasting *kombu* seaweed in the oven. Grind the roasted sesame seeds and *kombu* together, and add the mixture to a grain dish as a condiment.)
- Shoyu and tamari. (These are varieties of soy sauce used in cooking; avoid them as a condiment at the table to prevent excess sodium intake. Purchase low-sodium natural tamari and shoyu.)
- Sunflower seeds (roasted).
- Turmeric, cumin, clove, and other spices.
- *Umeboshi* dressings. (These flavorful dressings include *Umeboshi* plum, a Japanese plum considered to be health promoting.)

Oils

Oil is liquid fat. Vegetable and fish oils — referred to as polyun-saturated and monounsaturated fats — lower blood cholesterol levels somewhat, but excessive use of such oils has been linked to cancer. Use of all oils should be minimized. Sauté food in oils two or three times per week, preferably using olive oil or sesame oil. For baking, use corn oil.

Snacks and Desserts

Use unrefined, natural foods as snacks. Avoid oily, sugared, or processed foods. Use whole grains as snacks for their fiber, vita-min, and mineral content. We recommend the following snacks:

- Air-popped popcorn.
- Fruit (fresh, dried, or cooked; preferably in season).
- Good-quality whole grain bread, preferably sourdough. (Avoid yeasted bread if you are susceptible to yeast infections.)
- Natural candies made without refined sugar, such as those with rice syrup, barley malt, and fruit juice sweeteners.
- Natural, unsweetened apple butters, jams, and other spreads.
- Puffed grains.
- Rice cakes.
- Seeds and nuts (in small amounts).

Menu Suggestions

Breakfast

- Brown rice, made with more water than dinner rice; leftover dinner rice can be reheated with water to make it wetter and looser for the morning meal; it can be mixed with millet, oats, or bulgur wheat.

- Miso soup with *wakame* seaweed and a variety of other vegetables, including onions, carrots, and scallions.
- Oatmeal mixed with one of these ingredients: bulgur wheat, millet, raisins, rice syrup, or occasionally *natto* miso. Raisins can be added to the oatmeal to make it sweeter. A small amount — less than a teaspoon — of rice syrup can be added as a sweetener on occasion, as well. Rice syrup contains more complex sugars than most sweeteners.

Lunch

Lunch should include one item in each of the following categories:

- A serving of whole grain: brown rice, millet, barley, whole wheat, or corn. (The serving could consist of the grain itself, or bread or pasta made from it.)
- A green vegetable. (Collard greens, kale, mustard greens, turnip greens, and broccoli are among the best.)
- A root vegetable or squash, or any other vegetable.
- A piece of fresh fruit, preferably in season.

Dinner

- A whole grain should form the focus of the meal. Brown rice can be eaten regularly, though other forms of grain, such as bulgur wheat, whole wheat noodles, buckwheat flatcakes, and whole grain breads, should be used as well. Rice can also be mixed with beans.
- A leafy green, such as collard greens, kale, mustard greens, or turnip greens, or some other green vegetable should be included.
- A root vegetable or squash, or one of each — they can be

cooked together (perhaps acorn squash stuffed with carrots). Serve a yellow vegetable four to seven times per week.

- A bean, such as lentils, kidney beans, or fava beans, can form a separate dish or be mixed with grains or vegetables.
- Small servings (three ounces) of fish can form a side dish, but whole grains should constitute the center of the meal. White fish, such as haddock, cod, and flounder, is preferred because it is lower in fat than most red fish.
- Dessert should consist of fresh fruit, baked or raw, or a very occasional treat.

Recommendations for Obtaining Nutrients

Antioxidants

Beta-Carotene: There is no official recommended daily allowance (RDA) for beta-carotene, but we recommend ten to thirty milligrams per day; but fifty to one hundred milligrams is still safe if you need higher than normal levels of antioxidants. Rich sources for both vitamin A and beta-carotene are pumpkin, carrots, and cantaloupe.

Vitamin C: For vitamin C, the RDA is sixty milligrams. It is safe to use higher levels for the immunity-boosting effects. We recommend one hundred to four hundred milligrams per day. Higher amounts can cause health problems. Rich sources are peppers, broccoli, and strawberries. One medium green pepper will provide about 150 percent of the RDA.

Vitamin E: For vitamin E the RDA is eight milligrams for women and ten milligrams for men. For boosting immune responses and other healthful effects, you can safely use thirty to two hundred milligrams per day. Good sources are corn or safflower oil, nuts, and fatty fishes like salmon and mackerel. One ounce of sunflower seeds meets the RDA. Unlike the other antioxidants, which can be readily obtained from food, vitamin E may require supplementation.

■ ■ ■

See Chapter 4 for more complete information on these and other foods rich in antioxidants.

Minerals

Zinc: The recommended amount of zinc is fifteen milligrams for men and twelve milligrams for women. Too much zinc is harmful to the immune system. Good food sources include fortified breakfast cereals, oysters, and the dark meat of turkey. A serving of two eastern oysters more than meets the RDA.

Iron: The recommended amount of iron is ten milligrams for men and women and fifteen milligrams for women who menstruate. Iron too is harmful in excessive amounts, especially in combination with high levels of vitamin C. Good sources of iron include sardines, tofu, and millet. One half cup of tofu provides 44 percent of the RDA of iron for women.

Magnesium: The recommended amount of magnesium is 350 milligrams for men and 280 milligrams for women. Good sources of magnesium include tofu, spinach, oysters, and almonds. One ounce of almonds provides about a third of the RDA.

Fat

Eat low amounts of foods containing fats. The diet described here derives less than 20 percent of its total calories from fat (it includes more if you frequently eat animal foods). The health benefits of following a low-fat diet are substantial. Eat rich foods, such as steak and ice cream, on holidays or special occasions, but on a daily basis, follow the recommendations outlined in this section as closely as possible. The long-term pattern is the most important. After eating low-fat foods for a while, most people find they become less interested in high-fat foods. People with inflammatory diseases such as arthritis should try to increase the relative amount of fish oils in their diets because of its anti-inflammatory properties.

Herbs and Cancer-Fighting Foods

Include the following selections in your diet regularly:

- Chamomile tea
- Garlic
- Ginger (freshly grated)
- Green and black tea
- Licorice
- Shiitake and reishi mushrooms
- Turmeric, cumin, clove

To support your immune system during a bout with a cold or flu, use echinacea, astragalus, and other immunity-boosting herbs for three to seven days, and then stop.

Exercise

Make it a goal to exercise for thirty minutes a day, three to four days per week.

Your primary concern while exercising is doing what you enjoy. Walk in the woods, the park, along streets you like. Don't push yourself too hard or become a fanatic; overtraining is immunosuppressive. Moderate exercise is beneficial in many ways — to your immune system, your mind, your cardiovascular system, as a means of preventing major illness, as a way of fostering better sleep, and possibly as a way of extending your life. In any case, it will improve the quality of your life dramatically — as long as you enjoy and maintain a consistent program.

Body, Mind, and Spirit

The second half of the program involves ways of dealing with stress and making positive and supportive connections with those around us.

Positive Attitudes and Supportive Relationships

Here are six steps toward creating positive attitudes and supportive relationships.

1. Establish a relationship with a healer who supports your physical, mental, and spiritual health. Once you've found such a person, see him or her regularly. Many healers charge on a sliding scale. Barter if necessary. Priests, ministers, rabbis, and other clergy do not charge for their services. After you have connected with a healer, ask about support groups that he or she may know about or offer.

2. Join a support group, and stay with it. It can be part of your religious community; it can be a twelve-step program or a group with a specific theme or therapeutic approach, such as a men's or women's group, or a cancer-support group. Consider social clubs, or volunteer in your town or city at food pantries, soup kitchens, the Salvation Army, and other charitable organizations.

3. Establish friendships. This requires daring and flexibility, but it offers great rewards. Listen; be willing to be of service; be a friend in need; be gentle with others; avoid judgment and criticism.

4. Keep a journal, and write about your experiences and feelings as many days each week as you can.

5. Follow the diet recommended in this book. Especially concentrate on eating plenty of whole grains, vegetables, and fruits, all of which will boost your mood (grains are rich in complex carbohydrates that boost serotonin) and your immune system. The diet will also help you lose weight and make you look good.

6. Exercise four to five times per week for twenty to thirty minutes per exercise session. This will boost your mood and immunity and enhance your appearance.

Very Important: People who are clinically depressed need help. If you think of suicide, if your depression hangs on for weeks, if you have a poor appetite, or if you are not sleeping well, you need the help of a professional. Clinical depression is very common; more than 20 percent of the population will experience it at some time in their lives. Options for treatment include antidepressant medication and psychotherapy. Medications can be very effective, and some are not immunosuppressive.

There's no need to go it alone. Sometimes you need to discuss your problems with someone else to help get a broader perspective. Talk to a friend, a clergyman, or a professional counselor or therapist. Another choice is becoming part of a self-help group.

Conscious Living

Seek balance in your life, and avoid undermining your immune response by exposing yourself to poisons and negative influences. Take time to relax and enjoy yourself.

- Avoid recreational drugs.
- Limit alcohol intake to two drinks per day or less.
- Avoid exhaust fumes and environmental pollutants whenever possible.
- Protect yourself from overexposure to ultraviolet rays.

- Avoid immunity-depressing pharmaceuticals. (See Chapter 15 for a list of pharmaceutical drugs that depress the immune system.)
- Keep plenty of plants in your home. They clean the air and pump out oxygen.
- Be moderate in all things.
- Care for your body. Treat it as you would a loving friend. Give it good food, good medical care, exercise, an occasional therapeutic massage, and plenty of rest.
- Listen, as well as talk.
- Give and receive in friendship.
- Learn to be passive as well as aggressive, or vice versa if you tend to be passive.
- Release tension through deep breathing, exercise, meditation, and massage.
- Seek out small pleasures every day. Do something good for yourself, even if it's just ten minutes of walking, window shopping, or seeing a friend for lunch. Give yourself that present every day or several times per week as practice in maintaining balance.

A Week on the Program

Monday Morning

- *Breakfast.* Whole grain toast with sugarless jam, or toast with a slice of tofu (add a drop or two of tamari soy sauce); fresh fruit; tea: green tea, black tea, or chamomile or another herbal tea.
- *Exercise.* Twenty to thirty minutes of walking, aerobics, yoga, or stretching. *Note:* Exercise can be performed at any time in

the day. If it's easier for you to exercise at lunch or after dinner, do it then.

- *Spiritual practice.* Meditation, prayer, chanting, or sitting quietly in nature.

Monday Noon

- *Lunch.* Whole grain pasta sautéed in olive oil with onions, carrots, and collard greens.
- *Exercise.* A brisk walk.

Monday Evening

- *Dinner.* Brown rice with condiment; baked sweet potato; medley of greens, shiitake mushrooms, and carrots; pinto beans (cooked with *kombu* seaweed); and salad with balsamic vinegar dressing.
- *Exercise.* Evening walk or exercise at a health club.
- *Spiritual practice.* Meditate on the day. Do progressive relaxation.

Tuesday Morning

- *Breakfast.* Oatmeal with raisins, sweetened with rice syrup, if desired; green tea.
- *Exercise.* Twenty to thirty minutes of walking, yoga, stretching, or aerobics.
- *Spiritual practice.* Meditation, chanting, prayer, or sitting quietly in nature.

Tuesday Noon

- *Lunch.* Leftover grain from the previous night, or tabouli salad; asparagus.
- *Exercise.* A brisk walk.

Tuesday Evening

- *Dinner.* Lentil soup with leeks, rutabaga, and cauliflower, with miso and grated ginger added at the end of cooking; millet cooked with diced onions, carrots, garlic, dill, and a touch of sea salt; steamed mustard greens tossed with toasted white sesame seeds; beets cooked in apple juice with a little vinegar.
- *Spiritual practice.* Meditate on the day. Express gratitude for your life. Sing a happy song or listen to music.

Wednesday Morning

- *Breakfast.* Puffed cereal mixed with apple juice or soy milk; green tea, black tea, or a coffee derived from grains.
- *Exercise.* Ten to fifteen minutes of yoga, stretching, or a walk outside.
- *Spiritual practice.* Meditation, chanting, prayer, or sitting quietly in nature.

Wednesday Noon

- *Lunch.* Noodles in tamari broth with shiitake mushrooms, leeks, carrots, and onions; raw carrot and celery sticks.
- *Exercise.* A brisk walk.

Wednesday Evening

- *Dinner.* Baked salmon with mustard on the side; green beans with sliced almonds; roasted potatoes, coated in olive oil and sprinkled lightly with sea salt and pepper before cooking; sautéed onions, carrots, and cabbage.
- *Spiritual practice.* Call a friend or write a letter to someone you haven't been in touch with for a long time. Express appreciation for them.

Thursday Morning

- *Breakfast.* Cornmeal porridge flavored with brown rice syrup or maple syrup; green or black tea.
- *Exercise.* Ten to fifteen minutes of yoga, stretching, or aerobics, or a walk outside.
- *Spiritual practice.* Meditation, chanting, prayer, or sitting quietly in nature.

Thursday Noon

- *Lunch.* Stir-fried onions, carrots, broccoli, bamboo sprouts, mushrooms, and scallions, with grated ginger and shoyu; a few thin slices of whole grain bread.
- *Exercise.* A brisk walk.

Thursday Evening

- *Dinner.* Brown rice with condiments; baked winter squash; shiitake mushrooms sautéed in a sauce of water, barley malt, sake (wine), shoyu, and mustard; collard greens tossed with toasted sesame seeds.
- *Spiritual practice.* Progressive relaxation.

Friday Morning

- *Breakfast.* Rolled oats and Wheatena (with raisins, if desired); fresh fruit; green or black tea.
- *Exercise.* Ten to fifteen minutes of yoga, stretching, or aerobics, or a walk outside.
- *Spiritual practice.* Meditation, chanting, prayer, or sitting quietly in nature.

Friday Noon

- *Lunch.* Tofu sandwich with mustard, lettuce, Bermuda onion, shoyu sauce, balsamic vinegar, and grated ginger.
- *Exercise.* A brisk walk.

Friday Evening

- *Dinner.* Chickpea stew made with onions, carrots, and celery, seasoned with miso during last ten minutes of cooking, and garnished with dill and scallions; buckwheat noodles sautéed with onions and cabbage; turnips and rutabaga steamed together with a lemon-shoyu dressing; cucumber salad chilled in a bowl with salt for one hour, then drained and mixed with rice vinegar, toasted sesame oil, soy sauce, and maple syrup.
- *Spiritual practice.* Progressive relaxation, meditation, or journal writing.

Saturday Morning

- *Breakfast.* Boxed cereal from the natural foods store, eaten with apple juice or soy milk; fresh fruit; grain coffee or tea.
- *Exercise.* Ten to fifteen minutes of yoga, stretching, or aerobics, or a walk outside.
- *Spiritual practice.* Meditation, chanting, prayer, or sitting quietly in nature; attend synagogue (if desired).

Saturday Noon

- *Lunch.* Fish salad (mashed cooked white fish with chopped scallions, celery, and onion, mixed with tofu mayonnaise) sandwich on whole grain bread; salad with olive oil, lemon, and grated garlic.
- *Exercise.* A brisk walk.

Saturday Evening

- *Dinner.* Mushroom-barley soup with choice of vegetables and shoyu added at the end of cooking; pasta salad (diced carrots, peas, corn kernels, and whole grain noodles mixed with creamed tofu and white miso, and garnished with sesame seeds and scallions; broccoli sautéed in olive oil with garlic; *arame* seaweed with onions, carrots, toasted sesame seeds, and a dash of lemon juice and shoyu.
- *Spiritual practice.* Read the Bible, the Tao Teh Ching, the Lotus Sutra, or any other spiritually inspiring literature.

Sunday Morning

- *Breakfast.* Bagel with lox (avoid cream cheese); pancakes; homemade muffins or muffins purchased from a natural foods store; grain coffee.
- *Exercise.* Sleep late, and read the newspaper. You earned it.
- *Spiritual practice.* Attend church or temple (if desired). Think back on the past week, and allow yourself to feel gratitude for all your experiences.

Sunday Noon

- *Lunch.* A big salad with your favorite dressing.
- *Exercise.* Get together with friends and go for a bike ride, play volleyball, or organize a softball game.

Sunday Evening

- *Dinner.* Black beans with onions, carrots, red bell pepper, celery, garlic, black pepper, basil, and shoyu, placed in a taco shell and topped with salsa; brown rice fried with scallions and pieces of toasted *nori* seaweed; Swiss chard.

- *Spiritual practice.* Visit someone who needs cheering up.

■ ■ ■

This menu of choices can be adapted to suit your schedule or your whimsy. Its purpose is to show you that you can fit the entire program in any given week. Remember that most restaurants offer healthful choices, such as salads, steamed greens and carrots, and bread, if you are traveling or want a break from cooking at home. Many Asian or natural foods restaurants offer brown rice, vegetables, and even miso soup. With a little planning, much of your cooking can be done on the weekends or on one weeknight. A large pot of brown rice or beans will last for days in the refrigerator and can be reheated when you get home. Steaming greens and other vegetables can be done in three to seven minutes.

Once you get in the habit, boosting the immune system through this program can be as easy as your current lifestyle.

CHAPTER FIFTEEN

HIV, AIDS, and the Importance
of Immune System Boosters

AT THIS WRITING, there is no cure or vaccine against HIV and AIDS. That means that there are only two ways of protecting oneself from this dreaded disease: the first is prevention, which means abstaining from behaviors that put you at risk. The second is to maintain and, where possible, to boost your body's immune system. Of course, once a person is infected with HIV, prevention is no longer an option, which means that the only thing that stands between the infected person and AIDS that they can influence is the strength of the immune system. In this chapter, we want to address readers who are already infected with HIV and those who may already have AIDS. If you are in one or both of these groups, your single most important imperative is to keep your immune system strong. The stronger it is, the longer you can delay the onset of AIDS. Even after AIDS develops, the higher the level of CD4 cells, also referred to as T lymphocytes, the more likely that response to therapy will be good, and the odds for survival improved.

On average, it takes ten years after HIV infection for the immune system to fall to a dangerously low level of functioning. However, some people have been infected for more than ten years, have near-normal immune systems, and show no signs of illness. One of the remarkable characteristics of these people is that they tend to maintain higher levels of neutralizing antibodies — that is, antibodies that prevent the infection of new cells. They also have more T cells that target cells that contain HIV than people who progress more rapidly to AIDS. Such cells are referred to as anti-HIV cytotoxic T cells. Another characteristic of long-term survivors is that they actively take good care of themselves, which means that protecting their immune systems through appropriate lifestyle choices has been a priority for them.

It should be pointed out, however, that long-term survivors face just as powerful a disease as those who die soon after infection. Recent investigations show that most long-term survivors have equally virulent HIV strains as those who become ill, but nevertheless have somehow maintained good antiviral immunity. Many have never been treated with antiviral drugs, such as AZT. Presumably, their immune systems are the single most important factor in keeping them healthy.

The importance of a good immune response in preventing infection in the first place is still controversial. Other factors that are still unknown may play important roles in how the body deals with HIV. Also, some of the evidence suggests that a minority of people — certain infants and some adults with partners who are infected with HIV — may have the ability to totally clear HIV from their bodies after exposure. This group, however, represents a small number of people, and much more research must be done in order to understand this phenomenon. The vast majority of infected people have a single recourse, which is to take care of their immune systems.

HIV, AIDS, and the Destruction of the Immune System

Once it invades the human body, the human immunodeficiency virus undermines the immune system and leaves infected individuals vulnerable to attack by other infectious agents and to the development of certain cancers. HIV binds to the CD4 cell and to macrophages. (To put it more accurately, HIV binds to the CD4 molecule of T cells.) Over time, the CD4 cells (usually referred to as T helper cells) are destroyed, slowly at first, and then much faster as the immune system's ability to control the virus collapses. Eventually, virtually every aspect of immunity becomes weakened.

Although the structure of HIV and its life cycle are now understood in great detail, the mechanisms by which the immune system is destroyed are still largely hypothetical. It seems likely that an accumulation of several different actions leads to a final devastating effect.

Paradoxically, while the immune system is rapidly declining, certain other factors within the system become activated. These include CD8 cells and certain soluble factors, such as neopterin and beta$_2$-microglobulin. Unfortunately, these immune elements are counterproductive and are associated with a more rapid progression from HIV infection to AIDS.

This assault by HIV — causing the decline of protective elements and the rise of counterproductive factors — makes the virus so fiendish. Medical approaches that stimulate immunity run the risk of also encouraging the trend toward promoting virus production inside of infected cells. Thus it is important to carefully monitor HIV-infected people, because it is often very difficult to predict which treatment will actually work.

It is a tribute to the vigor of the immune system that opportunistic infections are uncommon before CD4 cell counts drop below two hundred cells per cubic millimeter of blood, which is far below a normal CD4 blood level of approximately one thousand cells per millimeter. Yet, even when the immune system falls below one quarter of its normal strength (approximately five hundred cells per millimeter), infections are usually kept in check.

This points directly to the need to maintain the immune system, and where possible, boost its strengths. The research community is finally starting to focus its efforts at understanding how medicine can support the immune system's fight against the virus, rather than concentrating all research efforts on finding a magic bullet cure for the disease (a struggle that has so far proved extremely frustrating but is finally yielding some encouraging results). While researchers continue the search for a cure and a vaccine, we must apply the existing knowledge of immune system boosters to support the body's efforts at maintaining immune strength. Fortunately, numerous studies show that many of the boosters we've been discussing can help HIV-infected people.

Here are some of the immunity-boosting tools that directly support the body's efforts in its fight against HIV.

Nutritional Boosters

Nutrition should be among the first immunity boosters adopted by HIV-infected people, especially since a substantial number develop a wasting syndrome or sustain periods of weight loss and are unable to regain the weight. In its severest form, the wasting syndrome can lead to death. Appetite stimulants such as megestrol acetate and dronabinol are of limited usefulness. They do help put on weight, but, unfortunately, that weight gain tends to be fat rather than the muscle tissue that has been lost.

Even those who do not suffer from wasting syndrome or gastrointestinal disorders can develop other nutritional and metabolic abnormalities. Many people with HIV experience elevations in resting energy metabolism, which means it takes more calories to maintain weight. As HIV progresses, the increase in metabolic rate causes weight loss and protein deficiency. Some of this elevation in metabolic rate is due to infections or intestinal disorders, but part of the weight loss is due to the rise in the inflammatory cytokines, tumor necrosis factor and interleukin-1, which lead to muscle breakdown and negative nitrogen balance.

Even without extensive weight loss, HIV-infected people suffer from numerous other nutrition-related problems, even in the early stages of the disease. A study of HIV-infected gay men in the Miami area indicated that 53 percent had low vitamin B_6 levels; 23 percent, low vitamin B_{12}; 26 percent, low riboflavin levels; and 10 percent, low vitamin C levels. Approximately 20 percent had low serum retinol (vitamin A) levels, and nearly 27 percent had low vitamin E (tocopherol) levels. Zinc levels were low or at the low end of normal in 50 percent of the HIV-positive subjects, and 63 percent had marginal copper levels.

Gay men who were not infected with HIV and served as controls had normal levels of all of these nutrients, with the exception of copper.

Given the importance of the majority of these nutrients to a healthy immune system, certainly low levels of these substances contribute to impaired immunity. In fact, several studies have shown that deficiencies of zinc, selenium, and vitamins B_6 and B_{12} do in fact influence immune system function in seropositive gay men.

Antioxidants: Immune System Boosters and Inhibitors of HIV

Vitamin A and Beta-Carotene

Antioxidant levels are often low in HIV-infected men. Since antioxidants seem to prevent HIV from replicating, low levels can speed up the disease process. Of the antioxidants, vitamin A and beta-carotene have recently received the most attention in HIV-positive populations. In the laboratory, vitamin A (retinoic acid, most often found in animal foods) inhibits HIV replication in macrophages, but it has little effect on T cells. Conversely, one study showed an opposite effect — that is, increases in HIV replication in retinoic-treated macrophages. In other laboratory research, retinoic acid also inhibited growth of Kaposi's sarcoma cells, and men with greater vitamin A intake are less likely to develop the sarcoma.

Beta-carotene was used as a supplement in two studies of HIV-infected people. One study administered 180 milligrams per day for four weeks and found that the percentage of CD4 counts went up during the period when beta-carotene intake was supplemented. No toxicity was observed. The other somewhat smaller study used lower doses of beta-carotene and was somewhat less successful. After administering a dose of 60 milligrams per day for four months, researchers found smaller increases in natural killer cells and activated lymphocytes, but no change in CD4 cell counts.

Although vitamin A deficiencies are generally uncommon in the United States, the risk of deficiency increases over two hundred times with HIV infection. In one study of men with AIDS who were not taking supplements, 22 percent had low levels of vitamin A in spite of the fact that the large majority had vitamin A intakes at or above the recommended daily allowance (RDA). Supplements seem to affect blood levels less effectively than food sources, however. Those who had food intakes of vitamin A of approximately two times the RDA were likely to have normal vitamin A blood levels. Beta-carotene levels were likely lowest in those with chronic diarrhea.

Vitamin A deficiency is associated with low CD4 cell levels and increased mortality in HIV-positive drug users. Also, CD4 counts were low in HIV-infected pregnant women with low beta-carotene or vitamin A levels. Overall, the levels of vitamin A and beta-carotene were about 40 percent lower in the HIV-infected women than in the control group.

Vitamin A deficiency also seems to be important in mother-to-child transmission of HIV. In a study of women in Malawi, those with vitamin A deficiencies were most likely to transmit the virus.

The rate of transmission ranged from 32 percent in those with the lowest vitamin A levels to 7 percent in those with the highest vitamin A levels.

Just as it is important not to become deficient in vitamin A, it is equally important not to take megadoses. Research has shown that among gay men, those consuming the highest levels of vitamin A were more likely to progress to AIDS than those with lower but adequate intake levels. Consistent with this research, other studies have shown that people who consume the lowest amount of vitamin A were more likely to progress to AIDS compared to those with moderate intakes.

Glutathione and Other Thiols

Other antioxidants are also important. German researchers reported that men with AIDS suffered from lower levels of the amino acid cysteine and the antioxidant glutathione in lymphocytes, monocytes, plasma, and fluids from the lungs. Both of these thiol compounds have important antioxidant functions; cysteine is the building block for glutathione. Glutathione is the most common antioxidant in cells.

Several studies have attempted to replenish low levels of cysteine and glutathione by giving the modified amino acid N-acetylcysteine (NAC). There are two potential benefits to this approach. One is an immunity-boosting effect, and the other is an antiviral effect. Lymphocytes require adequate levels of thiol compounds such as cysteine for optimal functioning. T cells utilize thiols in order to perform several functions, including T cell proliferation, cytotoxic activity, and responses to cytokines.

Cells from HIV-infected people die more rapidly, especially when activated by antigen. They die by a process known as apoptosis, or programmed cell death. Preliminary data from Luc Montanger's group at the Pasteur Institute in Paris suggest that giving

NAC reduces the amount of apoptosis seen in lymphocytes from HIV-infected subjects.

Thiol compounds, including NAC, also have been shown to inhibit HIV replication in infected cells, especially in cells stimulated with tumor necrosis factor. The level of NAC needed to enhance immunity is much lower than that needed for an antiviral effect. Other antioxidants, such as vitamin C, also inhibit HIV replication, perhaps in part by protecting cysteine from oxidation. Even at the high levels needed to inhibit HIV replication, NAC has low toxicity. NAC can be bought at health food stores and should be stored in the refrigerator.

In animal studies using mice with AIDS (MAIDS), long-term feeding of vitamin E slowed the development of abnormalities in cytokine production. Mice infected with the MAIDS virus overproduce interleukin-4 and underproduce interleukin-2; this is similar to conditions in some people with AIDS. This pattern of cytokine production favors the production of antibodies over the development of cell-mediated immunity. It has been suggested that this pattern partially explains why HIV-infected people have an inadequate immune response to the virus. Vitamin E helped correct this imbalance in mice and perhaps will do so in humans.

Recommendations

Antioxidants are probably the most important of the immunity-boosting nutrients. HIV-infected people, including those with AIDS, tend to show low levels of antioxidants. We recommend that you increase your intake of all dietary antioxidants above the RDA, but don't take megadoses of vitamin A, which may actually cause a faster progression to AIDS. Eating foods rich in antioxidants is preferable to taking supplements, with the possible exception of vitamin E. Chapter 4 includes a list of foods that are rich sources of antioxidants. In general, HIV infection seems to increase the demand for antioxidants, so that one hundred to two hundred milligrams of vitamin E per day seems desirable.

Minerals

Zinc and Copper

Although mineral levels are often abnormal in HIV-infected people, they do not seem related to diet. A large multicenter study found that seropositive men who progressed to AIDS during a two-and-a-half-year follow-up were significantly more likely to have had low serum levels of zinc and elevated levels of copper compared to those who did not progress to AIDS. Unlike vitamin A, blood levels of these trace minerals did not correlate with the amount of such minerals in their diets. Therefore, it isn't clear whether the low level of zinc contributed to the clinical deterioration or whether it was a consequence of clinical progression. Copper levels tend to increase and zinc levels to decrease in response to infections and the production of cytokines.

Taking large amounts of zinc supplements is definitely not the answer to low zinc levels. Another study found a greater risk of progressing to AIDS when dietary intake of zinc was increased. This result further emphasizes the danger of using megadoses of nutrients. The same study found niacin intake was associated with a decreased risk of progression.

Selenium

Selenium levels are reported to be low in HIV-infected people and those with AIDS. Selenium is low even when there are no gastro-intestinal problems, which, when they do occur, can prohibit absorption of selenium and other nutrients. Selenium tends to be low in individuals who have low zinc levels, leaving them particularly vulnerable to the effects of oxidation.

Iron

One study suggests that supplements containing thirty milligrams of iron may shorten survival in men with AIDS.

Recommendations

Avoid taking megadoses of zinc, even if zinc levels are low. Remember that in general, zinc levels that are too high are as immunosuppressive as levels that are too low. Also, for those infected with HIV, low levels of zinc cannot be corrected by taking more zinc, since the cause of low zinc has more to do with the way HIV changes the body than with eating too little zinc.

Eat foods that are rich in zinc, such as fortified cereals, beans, whole wheat and other grains, and shellfish, and maintain the RDA. If you decide to take zinc supplements, take low doses.

Avoid high doses of iron supplementation unless specifically prescribed.

Fat

Little is known about the effect of fats on HIV and AIDS. The literature suggests that calorie restriction and fish oils may be beneficial, but these reports need further study.

Weight Loss

Weight loss is a serious problem for many HIV-infected people. For some, weight loss is triggered by their inability to absorb fats. For people with this problem, dietary supplements that contain fats in simple form that are easily absorbed may be helpful in maintaining weight.

Recommendations

Keep fat intake low with the exception of fish oils, but make sure you are getting enough calories. If you are losing weight, discuss the possible causes with your physician, and begin the use of supplements. Chapter 6 lists the fat contents of selected foods.

General Recommendations for Nutrition

Get a blood nutritional analysis. Find out what nutrients are low and what the options are for improvement. It is clear from the studies cited that HIV infection creates additional nutritional demands, and the standard RDA for vitamins and minerals may not be sufficient to support the stressed immune system. Supplement where necessary, but avoid megadoses of all nutrients. Also, the increased metabolic rate that often accompanies HIV infection may require an increase in calorie intake to maintain weight.

Herbs and Botanical Preparations

Given the general lack of effective drugs against HIV, it is reasonable to explore all possibilities, including alternative medicines. In developing countries, traditional healers use various botanical preparations to treat HIV. Certain Chinese herbs and Ayurvedic medicines have been tested for anti-HIV activities, and some have resulted in positive reports. Perhaps the first to gain attention in this country was compound Q, also known as tricosanthin. It shows antiretroviral activity in vitro. In trials in HIV-infected volunteers, it caused transient decreases in levels of the viral protein p24 and decreases in beta$_2$-microglobulin, compounds that are associated with activation of HIV. It also improved immune system function and led to weight gain in people in the early stages of HIV infection. Unfortunately, it also seemed to have neurological toxicity, and several deaths were associated with its use.

Curcumin, found in turmeric, has shown anti-HIV activity in

the laboratory (in vitro) and is being tested on volunteers in community-based trials.

Other herbal or botanical derivatives have been shown to inhibit HIV replication in laboratory cell cultures. These include bioflavonoids isolated from *Chrysanthemum morifolium, Epimedium grandiflora, Viola yedoensis, Arctium lappa,* and *Glycyrrhiza uralensi;* dehydroandrographolide succinic acid monoester from the Chinese herb *Andrographis paniculata,* trioxanes from artemisinin *(qinghaosu);* novel alkaloids from the sponge *Batzella* sp.; and cucurbitacin-F from *Cowania mexicana.*

Carrageenan, a sulfated polysaccharide from red seaweed, is also being considered to prevent attachment of HIV to the genital tract epithelial cells. In a study of only two patients with HIV, long-term administration of a Chinese herbal medication, BG-104, was reported to restore plasma superoxide scavenging activity and to keep CD4 cell counts stable.

Polyphenols derived from tea have shown anti-HIV activity in the laboratory.

Mulberry seeds and roots contain 1-deoxynojirimycin, which has anti-HIV activity but also induces weight loss, which makes it problematic.

In laboratory studies, garlic has inhibited the growth of *Mycobacterium avium* complex, a common infection in AIDS. An extract from *Ginkgo biloba* leaves reportedly is active against *Pneumocystis carinii.*

Recommendations

Botanical derivatives may be useful but need more testing before they can be specifically recommended. If you do use herbal preparations, let your physician know. Some of the side effects of the herbs, such as diarrhea, headaches, and nausea, mimic some of the symptoms of HIV-related disease and of prescribed medications.

Psychological Factors

Given the connection between the mind and the immune system, it seems plausible that one's mental state or psychological makeup could affect progression of HIV. Evidence backing up this assumption exists, but it is not as simple as many seem to believe. There is little evidence that stress causes progression of the illness. The lack of evidence may be because the gay men who have been studied are remarkably resilient in dealing with HIV infection. Discovering that one is seropositive is enormously stressful, but there appears to be a rapid adjustment. The development of symptoms is also highly stressful. Yet, men who are symptomatic but have not yet developed AIDS are found to be more anxious and more depressed than men with AIDS. Overall levels of clinical depression or anxiety disorders are no more common among HIV-infected men at any stage than they are in the general population. In fact, the strongest predictor of mental illness for men with AIDS is a previous history of mental illness.

Benefits of Active, Healthful Coping

Staying in control and having a positive attitude do seem to have a positive effect on immunity, however. In a study at UCLA, scientists studied the effects of several different types of coping strategies, termed active-behavioral, active-cognitive, and avoidance for their effects on mood (including depression and anxiety) and self-reported health. Those using an active-behavioral coping style had lower levels of depression and anxiety and higher levels of social support, and they felt healthier. The active-positive style included measures such as taking more vitamins and eating healthy food, getting involved in political activities related to the illness, and enjoying everyday pleasures, events, and experiences more than they were previously enjoyed. Such an approach is also more commonly used by long-term survivors of HIV.

In contrast, the two coping strategies most associated with

high levels of depression and anxiety were avoidance and a passive-cognitive style. Avoidance included behaviors such as no longer associating with people, smoking, and increased use of drugs. Passive-cognitive style included daydreaming about better times and thinking about how things could have been done differently. It is hard to tell if the active approach is good because people ended up feeling less depressed or anxious, or because they were taking better care of themselves. Perhaps it was both.

In a Miami study, active coping, characterized as confident and forceful, was associated with improved natural killer cell activity. The researchers also looked for the effects of smoking, alcohol, drug use, and several nutritional factors on natural killer cell activity. Those with a history of smoking were associated with lower activity. Those with a history of eating foods rich in vitamin A (retinol) and omega-3 polyunsaturated fatty acids were associated with higher natural killer cell activity.

It is hard to know the significance of this study because natural killer cells do not appear to be important in the fight against HIV.

Depression and the Progression of the Disease

Perhaps because levels of depression tend to be so low in HIV-infected people, it has been difficult to consistently detect a relationship between depression and CD4 cell counts. CD4 cell counts are an ambiguous measure in HIV-infected people because the decline in CD4 can be seen both as a cause of the progression of the illness and as the result of such a progression.

Two large studies recently found that depressed gay men tended to have lower CD4 counts. The studies followed men from five to eight years. One found that depressed subjects had lower CD4 counts and more symptoms of disease. Unfortunately, it wasn't possible to tell if men were sicker because they were depressed or depressed because they were sicker. The other study found that CD4 cells dropped faster in men who were initially depressed, suggesting that perhaps depression led to a worsening of health. The magnitude of the effects was quite small, and other studies have found no similar effect.

Another study from UCLA found a fatalistic attitude toward bereavement went along with a decline in CD4 counts, a drop in overall immune response to antigens, and an increase in neopterin and beta$_2$-microglobulin, both measures of immune activation in response to the spread of HIV. Consistent with these findings was the fact that those with high fatalism scores were more likely to have a shorter survival time by nine months than those with low fatalism scores. Differences in use of AZT, initial CD4 values, psychological distress, smoking, and alcohol or drug use could not account for the different outcomes based on relative degree of fatalism. These results echo those of women with breast cancer who reacted to their cancer diagnosis with a fighting spirit rather than a stoic acceptance, and survived longer.

The Miami group has conducted several studies examining the effects of behavioral interventions on immune responses. The researchers recruited gay men who had not been tested for HIV. One group of men exercised, while another participated in what the scientists referred to as cognitive behavioral stress-management training. Both groups participated in their respective programs for five weeks prior to HIV testing, and then continued practicing their programs for five weeks after testing. Men from both groups showed less distress upon notification that they were HIV-positive than those without training. Immune depression after such notification was also less severe than it was for those who had no training.

When followed for an additional two years, those subjects who were most distressed by notification or who had the highest levels of denial in response to notification were most likely to progress to symptomatic disease. The researchers also found that those who most conscientiously followed the stress reduction program were less likely to progress to AIDS. However, having merely gone through the training programs was not protective;

sincerely adopting the techniques into overall lifestyle made the difference. The stress-management training included learning relaxation techniques, developing assertiveness and other active coping skills, and becoming aware of stresses. These programs worked for subjects evidencing various degrees of fitness, alcohol use, sleep, or frequency of sexual activity.

An animal model confirms the potential influence of social support. In a simian model of AIDS, the disruption of social structure was associated with a faster disease progression, including more rapid loss of lymphocytes and weight, and shorter survival time.

Recommendations

Attitudes matter. Keep trying to maintain your health. You will benefit both in the short term and in the long run.

Exercise

There is some evidence that exercising may be beneficial. The Miami study showed that exercise buffers the physiological and immunological changes of severe acute stress. In general, exercise decreases depression and increases self-esteem. People who are psychologically more hardy are also more likely to use exercise programs. Also, long-term survivors with AIDS generally participate in physical fitness programs. But aerobic fitness per se does not protect against progression. It could be that the mood-boosting effects of exercise are as important as the physical effects.

Recommendations

A regular program of exercise, even thirty minutes of brisk walking three days per week, will make you feel better and may have a positive impact on your immune system. Follow the recommendations in Chapter 8.

Harmful Behaviors

As would be expected, smoking and other harmful behaviors have a negative impact on the immune system.

However, the initial studies suggested at first that smoking might be beneficial. In several studies of large groups, the number of CD4 counts were found to be higher in seropositive men who smoked compared to those who didn't. The difference was gradually lost within two to three years following seroconversion. One study also showed that a protein associated with HIV progression, serum beta$_2$-microglobulin, was also elevated in smokers, suggesting that the increase in CD4 cells may be a temporary consequence of HIV activation, brought on by smoking. This would suggest that, rather than being helpful, the increase in CD4 cells may cause harm.

In another study, this interpretation was supported by the finding that smokers were more likely to have detectable HIV in their lungs and were more likely to die than nonsmokers. The study found that 47 percent of smokers died during the course of the study, whereas only 29 percent of nonsmokers died. The smokers were more likely to develop PCP pneumonia than nonsmokers. Interleukin-1 and interleukin-6 production by macrophages in the lungs were suppressed in HIV-infected smokers.

HIV-Infected Women and Smoking

Smoking beyond the first trimester of pregnancy is associated with an increased risk of transmission of the disease from mother to child. Mothers with low CD4 counts who continued smoking were three times as likely to transmit HIV to their infants as nonsmokers. For reasons that are not understood, smoking is also associated with a greater likelihood of becoming infected with HIV in certain groups of women.

Psychoactive Recreational Drugs and Immune Response

In studies that followed subjects for periods of up to eighteen months, use of alcohol, marijuana, volatile nitrites, amphetamines, barbiturates, or opiates did not seem to decrease CD4 counts or increase progression to AIDS in gay or bisexual men. In general, alcohol use was moderate in this group, with only 20 percent having two or more drinks per day. Between 40 and 50 percent had used marijuana or volatile nitrites in the past week. Several other studies confirmed these results.

However, heavy use of intravenous drugs is associated with a faster loss of CD4 cells than in people who use drugs less frequently or have stopped altogether. A Swiss study found the relative risk of progression to AIDS over a period of sixteen months was 1.78 for those who continued to inject drugs, compared to 0.48 for the methadone treatment group and 0.66 for former drug users. Also, drug users who used marijuana, crack, or cocaine were more than twenty times as likely to develop bacterial pneumonia. In laboratory tests, isobutyl nitrite has inhibited tumor-killing immune function and is associated with higher incidence of Kaposi's sarcoma.

In spite of a lack of clinical evidence for harmful effects from alcohol or cocaine, several laboratory studies suggest a need for caution. Adding cocaine or morphine to cultures of cells increases HIV production. Alcohol use is a risk factor for becoming HIV-positive, as is cocaine, but at least part of the effect is presumed to come from increased risk taking under the influence of the drugs.

Radiation and HIV

Ultraviolet light can induce HIV production. It generates oxygen radicals that induce the nuclear factor NF-κB, which in turn activates production of HIV. Ultraviolet irradiation of mice caused an increased expression of HIV in the cells of the skin. People who are HIV-positive also have HIV-infected cells in their skin, which could be activated by ultraviolet radiation.

It is unknown how significant ultraviolet rays can be, but studies suggest that sunbathing may carry some risk.

■ ■ ■

HIV infection and AIDS challenge us to take control of our lives in new and courageous ways. Experimentation with exotic therapies always involves a risk, but today such experimentation is especially appealing because of our lack of knowledge of long-term effective treatments. We recommend that people use the immunity-boosting program described in this book, especially the information in this chapter, as the basis for a healthy lifestyle. If you consider other experimental therapies, first conduct a thorough investigation of the existing literature and consult your physician while you ponder your decision. Meanwhile, study the information on long-term survivors, many of whom are using the "soft" methods described in this book as the basis for their health and longevity.

References

Baum, M., L. Cassetti, P. Bonvehi, G. Shor-Posner, Y. Lu, and H. Sauberlich. "Inadequate Dietary Intake and Altered Nutritional Status in Early HIV-1 Infection." *Nutrition* 10 (January–February 1994): 16–20.

Baum, M., E. Mantero-Atienza, G. Shor-Posner, M. Fletcher, R. Morgan, C. Eisdorfer, H. Sauberlich, P. Cornwell, and R. Beach. "Association of Vitamin B$_6$ Status with Parameters of Immune Function in Early HIV-1 Infection." *Journal of Acquired Immune Deficiency Syndromes* 4 (November 1991): 1122–32.

Beach, R., E. Mantero-Atienza, G. Shor-Posner, J. Javier, J. Szapocznik, R. Morgan, H. Sauberlich, P. Cornwell, C. Eisdorfer, and M. Baum. "Specific Nutrient Abnormalities in Asymptomatic HIV-1 Infection." *AIDS* 6 (July 1992): 701–8.

Bourinbaiar, A., and S. Lee-Huang. "Potentiation of Anti-HIV Activity of Anti-Inflammatory Drugs, Dexamethasone and Indomethacin, by MAP30, the Antiviral Agent from Bitter Melon." *Biochemical and Biophysical Research Communications* 208 (February 1995): 779–85.

Burack, J., D. Barrett, R. Stall, M. Chesney, M. Ekstrand, and T. Coates. "Depressive Symptoms and CD4 Lymphocyte Decline Among HIV-Infected Men." *Journal of the American Medical Association* 270 (December 1, 1993): 2568–73.

Burns, D., S. Landesman, L. Muenz, R. Nugent, J. Goedert, H. Minkoff, J. Walsh, H. Mendez, A. Rubinstein, and A. Willoughby. "Cigarette Smoking, Premature Rupture of Membranes, and Vertical Transmission of HIV-1 Among Women with Low CD4+ Levels." *Journal of Acquired Immune Deficiency Syndromes* 7 (July 1994): 718–26.

Caiaffa, W., D. Vlahov, N. Graham, J. Astemborski, L. Solomon, K. Nelson, and A. Munoz. "Drug Smoking, *Pneumocystis carinii pneumonis,* and Immunosuppression Increase Risk of Bacterial Pneumonia in Human Immunodeficiency Virus-Seropositive Injection Drug Users." *American Journal of Respiratory & Critical Care Medicine* 150 (December 1994): 1493–98.

Corbeau, P., M. Haran, H. Binz, and C. Devaux. "Jacalin, a Lectin with Anti-HIV-1 Properties, and HIV-1 gp120 Envelope Protein Interact with Distinct Regions of the CD4 Molecule." *Molecular Immunology* 31 (June 1994): 569–75.

Deshpande, R., M. Khan, D. Bhat, and R. Navalkar. "Inhibition of *Mycobacterium avium* Complex Isolates from AIDS Patients by Garlic *(Allium satium)." *Journal of Antimicrobial Chemotherapy* 32 (December 1993): 623–26.

Eck, H., H. Gmunder, M. Hartmanj, D. Petzoldt, V. Daniel, and W. Droge. "Low Concentrations of Acid-Soluble Thiol (Cysteine) in the Blood Plasma of HIV-1 Infected Patients." *Biological Chemistry Hoppe-Seyler* 370 (February 1989): 101–8.

Fesen, M., Y. Pommier, F. Leteurtre, S. Hiroguchi, J. Yung, and K. Kohn.

"Inhibition of HIV-1 Integrase by Flavones, Caffeic Acid Phenethyl Ester (CAPE), and Related Compounds." *Biochemical Pharmacology* 48 (August 3, 1994): 595–608.

Goodkin, K., N. Blaney, D. Feaster, M. Fletcher, M. Baum, E. Mantero-Atienza, N. Klimas, C. Millon, J. Szapocznik, and C. Eisdorfer. "Active Coping Style Is Associated with Natural Killer Cell Cytotoxicity in Asymptomatic HIV-1 Seropositive Homosexual Men." *Journal of Psychosomatic Research* 36 (May 1992): 1–16.

Guo, W., P. Gill, and T. Antakly. "Inhibition of AIDS–Kaposi's Sarcoma Cell Proliferation Following Retinoic Acid Receptor Activation." *Cancer Research* 55 (February 15, 1995): 823–29.

Harakeh, S., A. Niedzwiecki, and R. Jariwalla. "Mechanistic Aspects of Ascorbate Inhibition of Human Immunodeficiency Virus." *Chemico-Biological Interactions* 91 (June 1994): 207–15.

Hashimoto, F., Y. Kashiwada, G. Nonaka, I. Nishioka, T. Nohara, L. Cosentino, and K. Lee. "Evaluation of Tea Polyphenols as Anti-HIV Agents." *Bioorganic & Medicinal Chemistry Letters* 6 (1996): 695–700.

Hu, C., K. Chen, Q. Shi, R. Kilkuskie, Y. Cheng, and K. Lee. "Anti-AIDS Agents. 10. Acacetin-7-O-beta-D-Galactopyranoside, an Anti-HIV Principle from *Chrysanthemum morifolium* and a Structure-Activity Correlation with Some Related Flavonoids." *Journal of Natural Products — Lloydia* 57 (January 1994): 42–51.

Ironson, G., A. Friedman, N. Klimas, M. Antoni, M. Fletcher, A. LaPierre, J. Simoneau, and N. Schneiderman. "Distress, Denial, and Low Adherence to Behavioral Interventions Predict Faster Disease Progression in HIV-1 Infected Gay Men." *International Journal of Behavioral Medicine* 1 (1994): 90–105.

Jacobus, D. "Randomization to Iron Supplementation of Patients with Advanced Human Immunodeficiency Disease — an Inadvertent but Controlled Study with Results Important for Patient Care." *Journal of Infectious Diseases* 173 (April 1996): 1044–45.

Karter, D., A. Karter, R. Yarrish, C. Patterson, P. Kass, J. Nord, and J. Kislak. "Vitamin A Deficiency in Non-Vitamin-Supplemented Patients with AIDS: A Cross-Sectional Study." *Journal of AIDS and Human Retrovirology* 8 (February 1, 1995): 199–203.

Kemeny, M. "Stressful Events, Psychological Responses, and Progression of HIV Infection." In *Handbook of Human Stress and Immunity,* edited by R. Glaser and J. Kiecolt-Glaser. San Diego: Academic Press, 1994.

Lyketsos, C., D. Hoover, M. Guccione, W. Senterfitt, M. Dew, J. Wesch, M. Vanraden, G. Treisman, and H. Morgenstern. "Depressive Symptoms as Predictors of Medical Outcomes in HIV Infection." *Journal of the American Medical Association* 270 (December 1, 1993): 2563–67.

Mazumder, A., K. Raghavan, J. Weinstein, K. Kohn, and Y. Pommier. "Inhibition of Human Immunodeficiency Virus Type-1 Integrase by Curcumin." *Biochemical Pharmacology* 49 (August 1995): 1165–70.

Mihm, S., J. Ennen, U. Pessara, R. Kurth, and W. Droge. "Inhibition of HIV-1 Replication and NF-κB Activity by Cysteine and Cysteine Derivatives." *AIDS* 5 (May 1991): 497–503.

Namir, S., D. Wolcott, F. Fawzy, and M. Alumbaugh. "Coping with AIDS: Psychological and Health Implications." *Journal of Applied Social Psychology* 17 (March 1987): 309–28.

Schrauzer, G., and J. Sacher. "Selenium in the Maintenance and Therapy of HIV-Infected Patients." *Chemico-Biological Interactions* 91 (June 1994): 199–205.

Semba, R., P. Miotto, J. Chiphangwi, A. Saah, J. Canner, G. Dallabetta, and D. Hoover. "Maternal Vitamin A Deficiency and Mother-to-Child Transmission of AIDS." *Lancet* 343 (June 25, 1994): 1593–97.

Solomon, G., D. Benton, J. Harker, B. Bonavida, and M. Fletcher. "Prolonged Asymptomatic States in HIV-Seropositive Persons with 50 CD4+ T cells/mm^3: Preliminary Findings." *Journal of Acquired Immune Deficiency Syndromes* 6 (October 1993): 1172.

Tang, A., N. Graham, A. Kirby, L. McCall, W. Willett, and A. Saah. "Dietary Micronutrient Intake and Risk for Progression to Acquired Immunodeficiency Syndrome (AIDS) in Human Immunodeficiency Virus Type 1 (HIV-1)–Infected Homosexual Men." *American Journal of Epidemiology* 138 (November 1993): 937–51.

Twigg, H., D. Soliman, and B. Spain. "Impaired Alveolar Macrophage Accessory Cell Function and Reduced Incidence of Lymphocytic

Alveolitis in HIV-Infected Patients Who Smoke." *AIDS* 8 (May 1994): 611–18.

Ullrich, R., T. Schneider, W. Heisse, W. Schmidt, R. Averdunk, E. Riecken, and M. Zeitz. "Serum Carotene Deficiency in HIV-Infected Patients." *AIDS* 8 (May 1994): 661–65.

Vicenzi, E., and G. Poli. "Ultraviolet Irradiation and Cytokines as Regulators of HIV Latency and Expression." *Chemico-Biological Interactions* 91 (June 1994): 101–9.

Wang, Y., D. Huang, B. Liang, and R. Watson. "Nutritional Status and Immune Responses in Mice with Murine AIDS Are Normalized by Vitamin E Supplementation." *Journal of Nutrition* 124 (October 1994): 2024–32.

PART III

Scientific Evidence and Immune System Boosters

CHAPTER SIXTEEN

Antioxidants and the Science

S CIENTISTS NOW BELIEVE that antioxidants not only stave off illness and improve health but may also prolong life, in part because antioxidants prevent oxidative damage to the body's DNA. Oxidation is a major contributor to heart disease, inflammatory diseases such as arthritis, and cataract formation.

Oxidation and the Immune System

Oxidation harms your immune system largely by interfering with the delicate communication that takes place between the cell's receptors at its surface and its nucleus. When that occurs, the ability of the immune cell to recognize antigens is weakened, which can prevent the cell from identifying and dealing with bacteria, viruses, and even cancer cells. Oxidation also reduces the multiplication of T cells and B cells, natural killer cell activity, and production of antibodies, all of which are essential to mounting an effective defense against any infection. Oxidants can, however, induce inflammatory cytokines. Antioxidants help to protect the cell's membrane from the destructive effects of oxidants. They also boost the number of immune cells and increase the production of cytokines, the chemical messengers that facilitate communication within the immune system.

Arthritis

The chronic inflammation associated with arthritis boosts free radical production, which in turn promotes the disease and its painful symptoms. Unfortunately, inflammation is caused in part by the immune system's response to self-antigens present in the arthritic joints. The result is that the immune system, in the normal course of doing its job, makes things worse, in part by producing oxidants. Research has shown that people with chronic inflammation due to arthritis have low levels of antioxidants in their bloodstreams, and in fact have low levels of antioxidants even before symptoms appear. This is also true of people with inflammatory bowel disease. This makes antioxidants all the more important in the treatment of these diseases.

The Effects of Antioxidants

Here's a closer look at what individual antioxidants do for you and your immune system.

Beta-Carotene

Beta-carotene (the vegetable form of vitamin A) boosts your immune system in a number of ways. Studies have shown that it increases the number of CD4 and natural killer cells. It also boosts production of certain cytokines, especially interleukin-2, which stimulates T cell proliferation and function. However, some reports indicate that retinoids like beta-carotene can weaken killing by macrophages. This could become a problem for killing cancer cells, as some recent studies suggest.

Beta-carotene has been shown to strengthen the immune system's effort against *Candida albicans,* the most common cause of yeast infections. In developing countries where vitamin A deficiencies are common, vitamin A has been shown to dramatically reduce infections, particularly those of the intestines and lungs, and to reduce the death rate of children. In this country, vitamin A deficiencies are uncommon, but certain groups more frequently have low levels of beta-carotene or vitamin A. These include the elderly, menopausal women, smokers, asthma sufferers, and people getting chemotherapy for cancer.

Beta-Carotene and Heart Disease

Scientists at Brigham and Women's Hospital in Boston reported that men with a history of cardiovascular disease who took supplements of beta-carotene had approximately half the risk of heart attack, stroke, and death due to heart disease than those who didn't consume regular amounts of this immune system booster. The men in the study consumed fifty milligrams of beta-carotene every other day, an amount easily obtained from your diet.

A study of ninety thousand female nurses followed over eight years indicated that those nurses who ate regular amounts of fruits and vegetables rich in beta-carotene (the nurses got fifteen to twenty milligrams of beta-carotene per day from their diets) had 40 percent fewer heart attacks and strokes than controls who did not eat foods rich in this nutrient.

Beta-carotene is only one of hundreds of chemicals in the carotenoid family, not all of which have vitamin A activity. Several recent studies raise the possibility that the focus on beta-carotene has been too narrow and that other carotenoids, or combinations of carotenoids, may be more important than beta-carotene alone in preventing disease. Less is known about these other carotenoids, which are often found together with beta-carotene in food. Lycopene, for instance, is another potentially important carotenoid. It is abundant in tomatoes and seems to protect against cancer. Beta-carotene may be just the tip of the iceberg, and the scientific emphasis upon beta-carotene as a singular therapeutic agent may have caused researchers to miss the larger picture. Studies suggest that the unique shapes and properties of the various carotenoids help to deliver them to different locations in the body. It could very well be that carotenoids are far more important when they act together than when any single one acts alone.

Several recent studies have raised some concerns about beta-carotene as a cancer preventive and even suggest that people who use beta-carotene supplements may have a slightly greater chance of getting certain cancers. In one such study, first published in the *New England Journal of Medicine* and updated in the *American Journal of Clinical Nutrition,* men between the ages of fifty and sixty-nine who had been lifelong smokers were given fifty milligrams of vitamin E and twenty milligrams of beta-carotene per day. The study found that supplements of these two vitamins did not protect the men from lung cancer. In fact, those who took the beta-carotene supplements had a slightly increased risk of lung cancer as well as stomach cancer and prostate cancer. This finding is consistent with reports of less effective killing by macrophages exposed to retinoids.

But in an apparent paradox, results from the control group for this study — men who got no supplementation — showed that those with higher blood levels of both beta-carotene and vitamin E had the lowest levels of lung cancer, whereas those who had the lowest blood levels of beta-carotene and vitamin E had the highest rates of lung cancer. One way to interpret the paradox is to assume that supplementation is inferior to food as a source of vitamins, especially antioxidants. The scientists who conducted this study concluded that "it is better to obtain nutritionally active substances such as vitamin E and beta-carotene from a grocery store than from a pharmacy."

Similarly, in another study, death from all causes was lowest in those who had the highest initial concentration of beta-carotene in their blood when followed over an average of eight years. Conversely, those with the lowest beta-carotene levels were most likely to die, but taking beta-carotene in pill form had no effect on mortality.

Vitamin C

Vitamin C, which is water-soluble, works together with vitamins A and E, which are fat-soluble. Optimal levels of vitamin C — amounts between one hundred and four hundred milligrams per day — cause lymphocytes to react with greater vigor in the face of an antigen. Increased intake of vitamin C significantly boosts blood levels of the major antibodies IgG and IgM. Vitamin C stimulates natural killer cell activity and production of interferon, a chemical messenger that triggers a stronger immune response against viruses and some cancer cells. It also contributes to the health and vitality of macrophages.

Among its many useful immune effects, vitamin C seems to act like an antihistamine. Histamine is a chemical released from cells particularly during allergic reactions; it causes swelling and promotes inflammation. It is largely responsible for the symptoms of hay fever. Some reports note that vitamin C can reduce the symptoms of hay fever and arthritis.

The Nobel laureate Linus Pauling championed vitamin C as a preventive for the common cold. The evidence to date only partly supports that claim. An analysis that reviewed the results of twenty-one studies concluded that one gram per day of vitamin C could reduce the severity and duration of the common cold by 23 percent. It is still uncertain whether vitamin C reduces the frequency of colds. Vitamin C has also been shown to decrease the severity of respiratory infections in hospitalized elderly patients when doses of two hundred milligrams were taken daily.

A recent study indicates that the level of vitamin C in lymphocytes and in the blood reaches a plateau when people consume two hundred to four hundred milligrams per day. Higher levels of consumption did not deliver more vitamin C into the bloodstream.

Vitamin E

Vitamin E is especially protective against the normal age-related decline of the immune system. Also known as tocopherol, vitamin E is essential to the maintenance of normal metabolism and immune function. It also reduces muscle damage, especially after exercise. Vitamin E deficiencies in humans are associated with impaired T cell activity and increased incidence of infectious diseases.

Feeding high levels of vitamin E (fifty to nine hundred milligrams per day) to subjects increased the ability of their lymphocytes to multiply in response to stimulation. Vitamin E has also been shown to increase production of interleukin-2. It stimulates the activity of natural killer cells that seek out and destroy viruses and cancer cells. It can also boost phagocytic activity of granulocytes. Studies have shown that four hundred milligrams of vitamin E taken daily by glutathione-deficient infants boosted their phagocytic activity significantly.

While vitamin E boosts the reaction of immune cells to infections, it also seems to mitigate the toxic side effects of activities of the immune system. For example, immune cells produce less peroxide and prostaglandins — both of which cause tissues to become inflamed — after they phagocytize (or consume) a pathogen. By limiting inflammation, the immune system is able to work more efficiently and apparently against less self-created resistance.

Studies done at Tufts University have shown that vitamin E causes lymphocytes to react more vigorously against a TB antigen. These cells also proliferate more rapidly in the face of an antigen.

Not only does vitamin E cause a short-term improvement of immune function, but also research has shown that after six months of vitamin E supplementation — at two hundred milligrams per day — the antioxidant resulted in sustained and dramatic improvement of the immune response.

Vitamin E and Cancer

Vitamin E intake has been correlated with lower incidence and death rate from cancer. In a study of Chinese, supplementation with vitamin E at two times the RDA was associated with lower cancer rates, particularly cancer of the stomach. The RDA for vitamin E is ten milligrams per day. Two or three times that amount can be obtained from dietary sources alone. The differences in cancer rates among those consuming at least ten to twenty milligrams of vitamin E per day could be seen within two years.

Vitamin E and Heart Disease

In addition to the ability of vitamin E to prevent the development of heart disease, it can also apparently slow the progress in those who already have symptoms of disease. A study reported that vitamin E could slow artery obstruction in men who had previously had artery bypass surgery. Using serial angiography to measure the size of the artery opening, they found that men who took one hundred or more milligrams of vitamin E per day had less clogging of their blood vessels over the two years of taking the vitamin.

In a study of 34,486 postmenopausal women, vitamin E intake from food was associated with a reduced risk of death from heart disease, whereas vitamins A and C had no effect. Women eating the most vitamin E reduced their risk of death from heart disease to 0.42, compared to those who consumed the least vitamin E.

Remember, antioxidants have far more powerful health benefits when they are consumed together, rather than individually. Taking individual antioxidants in pill form prevents you from getting the variety of antioxidants present in food. In addition, vegetable foods contain other nutrients that offer specific protection against cancer. An evaluation of the antioxidant capacity of fruits resulted in this list, which gives them in order from highest to lowest capacity: strawberries, plums, oranges, red grapes, kiwi fruit, pink grapefruit, white grapes, bananas, apples, tomatoes, pears, honeydew melon. For fruit juices, the order was grape, grapefruit, tomato, orange, apple.

Supplements of beta-carotene or vitamin A may be needed by patients dealing with cancer, hepatitis, chronic infections, or kidney or prostate disease, in which large amounts of vitamin A are often excreted.

However, dangers result from taking excessive amounts of antioxidants; the body does in fact need a certain amount of oxidation for cells to maintain themselves and produce energy. High intake of beta-carotene is not thought to be toxic, although people who take lots of it often begin to turn orange. Vitamin A in excess can pose a problem; hazards include headaches, vomiting, nausea, weight loss, fatigue, hair loss, dry skin, and liver damage. Six thousand micrograms per day may cause birth defects if taken by pregnant women.

Smoking decreases absorption of vitamin C so that intake should increase by roughly twenty-five milligrams per pack per day. Even passive smoke lowers antioxidant levels in the blood, for instance, in the children of smokers. Heavy drinkers and those who use a lot of aspirin may also want to increase intake, but even so it seems that dietary sources, which are so abundant, should be able to supply the extra need without use of supplements.

Hazards related to megadoses of vitamin C include bladder

and kidney stones, urinary tract irritation, and cramps and diarrhea. In people with high iron stores, vitamin C acts as an oxidant — the opposite effect intended for an antioxidant — and it can be dangerous for people with sickle cell anemia. Also, the body adjusts to high intake levels by increasing metabolism and excretion, so that when megadoses are stopped, normally adequate levels of intake can lead to vitamin C deficiency. Five hundred milligrams per day is suggested as the upper limit for daily supplementation.

Vitamin E supplements are needed in premature infants and people with malabsorption problems. Excess vitamin E is associated with lower thyroid levels, fatigue, weakness, blurred vision, and gastrointestinal problems. Vitamin E accumulates in the body, and long-term use at high levels may be excessive.

Bioflavonoids and Stroke

A study from the Netherlands of 552 men aged 50–69 years who were followed for 15 years found a substantially lower incidence of strokes in those with the highest consumption of bioflavonoids. The conclusion held up after taking into account consumption of fish, alcohol, and other antioxidants. Black tea accounted for 70 percent of bioflavonoid intake in this cohort. The group with the fewest strokes were drinking more than four cups of tea a day on average.

References

Albanes, D., O. Heinonen, J. Huttunen, P. Taylor, J. Virtamo, B. Edwards, J. Haapakoski, M. Rautalahti, A. Hartman, J. Palmgren, and P. Greenwald. "Effect of Vitamin E and Beta-Carotene Supplements on Cancer Incidence in the Alpha-Tocopherol and Beta-Carotene Cancer Prevention Study." *American Journal of Clinical Nutrition* 62 (supplement 1995): S1427–30.

Alexander, M., H. Newmark, and R. Miller. "Oral Beta-Carotene Can Increase the Number of OKT4+ Cells in Human Blood." *Immunology Letters* 9 (1985): 221–24.

Ames, B., M. Shigenaga, and T. Hagen. "Oxidants, Antioxidants, and the Degenerative Diseases of Aging." *Proceedings of the National Academy of Sciences* 90 (September 1993): 7915–22.

Bendich, A. "Role of Antioxidants in the Maintenance of Immune Functions." In *Natural Antioxidants in Human Health and Disease,* vol. 4, edited by B. Frei. San Diego: Academic Press, 1994.

Blot, W., J. Li, P. Taylor, W. Guo, S. Dawsey, G. Wang, C. Yang, S. Zheng, M. Gail, G. Li, Y. Yu, B. Liu, J. Tangrea, Y. Sun, F. Liu, J. Fraumeni, Y. Zhang, and B. Li. "Nutrition Intervention Trials in Linxian, China — Supplementation with Specific Vitamin/Mineral Combinations, Cancer Incidence, and Disease-Specific Mortality in the General Population." *Journal of the National Cancer Institute* 85 (September 15, 1993): 1483–92.

Chandra, R. K. "Effects of Vitamin and Trace-Element Supplementation on Immune Responses Among the Elderly." *Lancet* 340 (November 7, 1992): 1124–27.

Chen, J., C. Geissler, B. Parpia, J. Li, and T. Campbell. "Antioxidant Status and Cancer Mortality in China." *International Journal of Epidemiology* 21 (April 1992): 625–35.

Cross, C., and B. Halliwell. "Nutrition and Human Disease: How Much Extra Vitamin C Might Smokers Need?" *Lancet* 341 (April 24, 1993): 1091.

Frei, B., L. England, and B. Ames. "Ascorbate Is an Outstanding Antioxidant in Human Blood Plasma." *Proceedings of the National Academy of Sciences* 86 (August 1989): 6377–81.

Gey, K., P. Puska, P. Jordan, and U. Moser. "Inverse Correlation Between Plasma Vitamin E and Mortality from Ischemic Heart Disease in Cross-Cultural Epidemiology." *American Journal of Clinical Nutrition* 53 (January 1991): 326S–34S.

Greenberg, E., J. Baron, M. Karagas, T. Stukel, D. Nierenberg, M. Stevens, J. Mandel, and R. Haile. "Mortality Associated with Low Plasma Concentration of Beta-Carotene and the Effect of Oral Supplementation." *Journal of the American Medical Association* (March 7, 1996): 699–703.

Heliovaara, M., P. Knekt, K. Aho, R. Aaran, G. Alfthan, and A. Aromaa. "Serum Antioxidants and Risk of Rheumatoid Arthritis." *Annals of the Rheumatic Diseases* 53 (January 1994): 51–53.

Hemila, H. "Does Vitamin C Alleviate the Symptoms of the Common Cold? — a Review of Current Evidence." *Scandinavian Journal of Infectious Diseases* 26 (January 1994): 1–6.

Hodis, H., W. Mack, L. LaBree, L. Cashin-Hemphill, A. Sevanian, R. Johnson, and S. Azen. "Serial Coronary Angiographic Evidence That Antioxidant Vitamin Intake Reduces Progression of Coronary Artery Atherosclerosis." *Journal of the American Medical Association* 273 (June 21, 1995): 1849–54.

Hunt, C., N. Chakravorty, G. Annon, N. Habibzadeh, and C. Schorah. "The Clinical Effects of Vitamin C Supplementation in Elderly Hospitalized Patients with Acute Respiratory Infections." *International Journal of Vitamin and Nutrition Research* 64 (1994): 212–19.

Keli, S., M. Hertog, E. Feskens, and D. Kromhout. "Dietary Flavonoids, Antioxidant Vitamins, and Incidence of Stroke: The Zutphen Study." *Archives of Internal Medicine* 156 (March 1996): 637–42.

Kornhauser, A., L. Lambert, W. Wamer, R. Wei, S. Lavu, and W. Timmer. "Antioxidants and Cancer Prevention in Vivo and in Vitro." In *Nutrition in Cancer Prevention and Treatment,* edited by K. Prasad. Totowa, N.J.: Humana Press, 1995.

Kushi, L., A. Folsom, R. Prineas, P. Mink, Y. Wu, and R. Bostick. "Dietary Antioxidant Vitamins and Death from Coronary Heart Disease in Postmenopausal Women." *New England Journal of Medicine* 334 (May 2, 1996): 1156–62.

Levine, M., C. Conry-Cantilena, Y. Wang, R. Welch, P. Washko, K. Dhariwal, J. Park, A. Lazarev, J. Graumlich, and J. King. "Vitamin C Pharmokinetics in Healthy Volunteers: Evidence for a Recommended Dietary Allowance." *Proceedings of the National Academy of Sciences* 93 (April 16, 1996): 3704–9.

Meydani, S., M. Barkland, S. Liu, M. Meydani, M. Miller, J. Cannon, F. Marrow, R. Rockilin, and J. Blumberg. "Vitamin E Supplementation Enhances Cell-Mediated Immunity in Healthy Elderly Subjects." *American Journal of Clinical Nutrition* 52 (September 1990): 557–63.

Meydani, S., M. Hayek, and L. Coleman. "Influence of Vitamins E and B_6 on Immune Response." *Annals of the New York Academy of Sciences* 669 (1992): 125–40.

Rimm, E., M. Stampfer, A. Ascherio, E. Giovannucci, G. Colditz, and W. Willet. "Vitamin E Consumption and the Risk of Coronary Heart Disease in Men." *New England Journal of Medicine* 328 (May 20, 1993): 1450–56.

Sommer, A. "Vitamin A, Infectious Disease, and Childhood Mortality: A 2c Solution?" *Journal of Infectious Diseases* 167 (1993): 1003–7.

Stampfer, M., C. Henneken, J. Manson, G. Colditz, B. Rosner, and W. Willet. "Vitamin E Consumption and the Risk of Coronary Heart Disease in Women." *New England Journal of Medicine* 328 (May 20, 1993): 1444–49.

Wang, H., G. Cao, and R. Prior. "Total Antioxidant Capacity of Fruits." *Journal of Agricultural and Food Chemistry* 44 (March 1996): 701–5.

CHAPTER SEVENTEEN

Minerals and the Science

METAL IONS ARE NEEDED throughout the body. They interact with proteins to help them function. Proteins have some flexibility in their shape but must be in a precise arrangement to function effectively. Proteins are synthesized as a linear array of amino acids. This string of amino acids is then arranged into a three-dimensional structure that looks like a tangled ball of yarn. The twists and turns are to some extent dictated by the sequence of the amino acids. Very often a metal ion will form a bridge between different loops of the protein and help it stabilize its shape in a form that allows it to function. The positive charges on the metal ion interact with negative charges on the protein. Different proteins require different ions to do this. Many use zinc; others use iron, magnesium, or copper. Zinc and copper, for instance, are needed for the functioning of the enzyme superoxide dismutase, an enzyme that destroys otherwise harmful oxidants. As noted in Chapter 5, the immune system is sensitive to dietary levels (both excesses and deficiencies) of a number of metals.

Zinc

Zinc is needed for both the development and function of T lymphocytes. Zinc is required in the thymus to help immature thymocytes develop into mature T cells. Zinc levels also influence mature CD4 cells after they leave the thymus. Without adequate zinc, these T lymphocytes are less responsive to a challenge. They don't divide as effectively in response to stimulation. Thus, zinc deficiency is associated with lower than normal numbers of T cells, particularly CD4 cells. Without a strong CD4 response, the overall immune reaction is weakened significantly, since it is the CD4 cell that directs and stimulates many other important members of the immune armamentarium. However, when zinc levels are normalized, the T cell response is also restored. Under certain circumstances, zinc by itself is sufficient to cause T lymphocytes to multiply without the presence of antigens.

T cells are not the only immune cells whose function is impaired by inadequate zinc. Natural killer cells are significantly less reactive. They are particularly important in the fight against tumor cells, and any decrease in their number or their aggressiveness could mean greater vulnerability to cancer. Also, natural killer cells are the first line of defense against viruses, so their lowered activity could mean greater susceptibility to viral infections. In addition, when zinc is low, B cells fail to produce adequate amounts of antibodies, which makes the immune response to bacteria less effective.

It is not surprising, then, that children with inadequate zinc in their bloodstreams have been shown to have significantly higher rates of infection than those with adequate zinc. In one study, thirty-two infants were divided into two groups, one supplemented with zinc, the other receiving placebo. Those who received the zinc had far fewer infections, gained more weight, and had higher blood levels of T cells and antibodies.

In another study, which examined the CD4 responses in children with Down syndrome, researchers found that CD4 cells did not multiply well in response to stimulation. Children with Down syndrome tend to have low levels of zinc. However, when the children were given supplements of zinc (twenty milligrams per kilogram of body weight per day) for two months, their proliferative response returned to normal and stayed normal for six months. The improved responses dropped off after zinc supplements were discontinued. Another study showed that children with Down syndrome had fewer infections when they were given zinc supplements, presumably because their immune function had improved.

Colds didn't last as long in a study of healthy adults who took zinc pills. The colds lasted for 4.9 days in the supplemented zinc group, versus 6.1 days for the lower zinc group. These differences in the length of colds occurred when zinc was taken before the cold began. However, zinc was also shown to be effective when taken a day after the cold began (4.3 days versus 9.2 days). Cold symptoms, such as cough, nasal drainage, and congestion, were lower among those who took additional zinc.

In animal studies, mice on low-zinc diets were less able to fight candidiasis and parasitic infections, partly because of an impaired ability to produce cytokines, and partly because of reduced killing by macrophages.

The developing immune system seems especially sensitive to low levels of zinc. In animal studies it was found that even marginal zinc deficiencies in a pregnant mother were responsible for long-lasting impairment in the offspring's immune responses. Again, it was mainly the T cell responses that were affected.

The Effects of Excess Zinc

Although zinc is clearly needed for optimal functioning of the immune system, excessive blood levels of zinc are harmful for the immune system. In one study, healthy men were fed three hundred milligrams of zinc per day for six weeks. (An average dietary intake of zinc is approximately ten to fifteen milligrams per day.) The researchers found that, just as with inadequate zinc, excessive zinc also depressed the T cell response to an antigen. Granulocyte function was also adversely affected.

Normal blood levels of zinc are one hundred micrograms per deciliter; blood levels of three hundred micrograms per deciliter or higher are associated with immune system impairment. As noted in Chapter 5, megadoses of zinc can also create gastrointestinal problems and are a danger to pregnant women.

The consumption of zinc-rich foods alone can cause T lymphocytes to proliferate and trigger B cells to secrete antibodies, especially if blood levels of zinc have been low before the introduction of zinc-rich foods. Once again, moderation is essential.

The people who most commonly have low zinc levels are intravenous drug abusers and alcoholics, especially alcoholics with cirrhosis of the liver. Other people at risk are patients with inflammatory bowel disease, adolescents, and the elderly. All three of these groups tend to follow narrow diets that may be inadequate in zinc. Convalescing adults experience higher than average demands for zinc when muscle tissue must be replaced. Zinc levels are also likely to be lower in people with severe arthritis. In this case the low blood levels are a result of the inflammation associated with arthritis and the production of cytokines such as interleukin-1, which cause zinc to be removed from the circulation. Here, the way to improve zinc levels is to reduce the inflammatory reaction.

Iron

Iron is another mineral that influences the immune system. But because cells of the immune system have extensive mechanisms to control their internal iron levels, they seem to be able to function normally over a fairly wide range of external iron levels. Lymphocytes get most of their iron bound to a plasma protein known as transferrin. When they need iron, they produce transferrin receptors, which they place on their surfaces to catch the plasma transferrin molecules and their attached iron ions. The cells do this when the level of iron within the cell becomes low, or when the cells are activated and are preparing to divide. Iron is needed for the function of ribonucleotide reductase, an enzyme that controls DNA synthesis. Iron is also needed for cellular respiration in the mitochondria, the intracellular organelles that carry out the cell's oxygen exchange. When iron levels are high in the cell, and when the cell has finished dividing, it begins to make another iron-binding protein called ferritin, which binds the excess iron and helps excrete it from the cell. T lymphocytes and natural killer cells do not have any detectable transferrin receptors unless they are activated. B lymphocytes, on the other hand, have low levels of transferrin receptors when they are resting, and they increase the number of these receptors when they are activated. Perhaps because of this difference, T cells are more sensitive to low levels of iron than are B cells. T cells proliferate less well in people with iron deficiency, and the helper T cells involved in inflammation seem more affected by low iron than the helper T cells involved in helping B cells make antibodies. As expected, then, antibody production is relatively normal even in iron-deficient individuals.

Iron deficiency in children occurs during periods of high growth rates and is most common in the second six months of the first year and again during the postpubertal growth phase. Iron deficiency anemia in adults is nearly always related to blood loss. Anemia is most often found in people over age fifty with hemorrhoids, peptic ulceration, hiatal hernia, diverticulosis, and chronic aspirin use. Heavy menstrual blood flow and pregnancy also can cause anemia. Iron deficiency weakens the immune system even before anemia develops.

The Effects of Excess Iron

Excess iron, like zinc, depresses immunity. The effects of excess iron on individual immune cells, however, are not as well understood. Macrophages mop up excess iron in tissues and the blood, which suggests that the immune system may be regulating the amount of iron in the bloodstream. This occurs especially when macrophages are cleaning up the debris in wounds.

Some people feel that supplementation of iron is associated with greater risk of dying of heart disease, but the data so far are inconclusive. Excessive levels of iron act as an oxidant, helping to transform LDL cholesterol into its more dangerous oxidized form. Vitamin C triggers the oxidation of iron, suggesting that those who take vitamin and mineral supplements may be at higher risk.

Additional hazards of excess iron include buildup of stores in the liver, the pancreas, and sometimes, the heart. Too much iron can interfere with zinc uptake and cause arrhythmias.

Magnesium

Clinical manifestations of magnesium deficiency include neuromuscular dysfunction (such as involuntary muscle contraction), convulsions, tremors, and muscle weakness; behavioral abnormalities such as anxiety, disorientation, confusion, and psychotic behavior; and cardiovascular abnormalities, particularly tachycardia. Low magnesium levels are associated with gastrointestinal disorders including chronic diarrhea and celiac disease; kidney disorders; alcoholism, with or without cirrhosis; and certain endocrine disorders such as hyper- or hypoparathyroidism, hyperthyroidism, and diabetes mellitus. Excess magnesium is associated with kidney failure, and magnesium may be slightly elevated by lithium therapy. Excess magnesium can lead to paralysis and respiratory failure.

References

Bronner, F., and J. Coburn, eds. *Disorders of Mineral Metabolism.* Vols. 1–3. San Diego: Academic Press, 1981.

Godfrey, J., B. Conant Sloane, D. Smith, J. Turco, N. Mercer, and N. Godfrey. "Zinc Gluconate and the Common Cold: A Controlled Clinical Study." *Journal of International Medical Research* 20 (June 20, 1992): 234–46.

Good, R., and E. Lorenz. "Nutrition and Cellular Immunity." *International Journal of Immunopharmacology* 14 (April 1992): 361–67.

Kemp, J. "The Role of Iron and Iron-Binding Proteins in Lymphocyte Physiology and Pathology." *Journal of Clinical Immunology* 13 (February 1993): 81–89.

Kumari, B., and R. K. Chandra. "Overnutrition and Immune Responses." *Nutrition Research* 13 (supplement 1, 1993): S3–S18.

Licastro, F., M. Chiricolo, E. Mocchegianni, N. Fabris, M. Zannoti, E. Beltrandi, R. Mancini, R. Parente, G. Arena, and M. Masi. "Oral Supplementation in Down Syndrome Subjects Decreased Infections and Normalized Some Humoral and Cellular Parameters." *Journal of Intellectual Disability Research* 38 (April 1994): 149–62.

McCoy, H., and M. Kenney. "Magnesium and Immune Function: Recent Findings." *Magnesium Research* 5 (December 1992): 281–93.

Mei, W., Z. Dong, B. Liao, and H. Xu. "Study of Immune Function of Cancer Patients Influenced by Supplemental Zinc or Selenium-Zinc Combination." *Biological Trace Element Research* 28 (January 1991): 11–19.

Prohaska, J., and O. Lukasewycz. "Effects of Copper Deficiency on the Immune System." *Advances in Experimental Medicine and Biology* 262 (1990): 123–43.

CHAPTER EIGHTEEN

A Low-Fat Diet and the Science

ALTHOUGH THE DRAWBACKS of fat have become well publicized, we all need a certain amount of fat to stay healthy. Cells of the immune system are particularly sensitive to both the amount and types of fat we eat. The cell membrane forms the boundary between the inside and outside of the cell. It consists of approximately half protein and half lipid, or fat. The composition of the fats in the membrane is influenced by diet. The more polyunsaturated fats we eat, the more polyunsaturated fats end up in the membrane. The lipid composition of the cell membrane affects the way the cell communicates with the world outside of it. It can influence both the recognition of and the response to dangers. Although polyunsaturated fats are generally recommended in preference to saturated fats to reduce the risk of heart disease, for the immune system, polyunsaturates are generally thought to be as bad if not worse than saturated fats. In some studies, increasing fat, particularly fish oils, is being attempted to dampen immunity and reduce inflammation.

A study published in *Clinical Immunology and Immunopathology* reported on the effects of three diets on women and their immune systems. All the women started on a high-fat diet, consisting of 41 percent fat, during which time their lymphocytes were tested for their ability to multiply after stimulation. Once this was done, the women were divided into two groups, each of which got diets lower in fat. One group received a diet containing 26 percent of its calories from fat, with 3 percent of that fat coming from polyunsaturated fats. The other group followed a diet containing 31 percent fat, of which 9.1 percent was from polyunsaturated fat. Once again, the lymphocytes were challenged to divide.

The scientists discovered that the lymphocytes responded far more vigorously when the women were eating one of the low-fat diets than they did while they were eating the high-fat diet. Women on the low-fat regimens also produced more complement in their blood. The study did not uncover any difference in immune response between the two low-fat diets; both boosted the immune system equally.

Natural killer cell activity is also suppressed by high levels of fat. In one study, researchers measured the natural killer cell activity of men on a high-fat diet (fat made up 40 percent of their total calories). Researchers then placed the same men on a low-fat diet (consisting of approximately 22 percent total fat) and found that the natural killer cell destruction of tumor cells doubled. When the men were returned to the high-fat diet, the vigor of natural killer cell activity was once again cut in half. Both this study and the one mentioned before were able to pinpoint the connection between fat and reduced immune function since each subject served as his own control. The use of this type of study rules out the influence of other lifestyle factors such as smoking or exercise, since these factors were unchanged over the duration of the study. When the scientists took calorie levels into account, they found that fat had an independent and deadening effect on natural killer cell effectiveness.

When macrophages metabolize fats, they produce prostaglandins, which suppress both macrophage and T cell functions, making them less responsive to the presence of an antigen. By forcing macrophages to produce more of these substances, fat turns the macrophages into immune-suppressor cells. Research has shown that polyunsaturated fats are especially effective at causing macrophages to produce prostaglandins. This is one way that excess consumption of polyunsaturated fats can depress immune function and make us more vulnerable to disease.

Some studies have shown that polyunsaturated fats decrease antibody production by B cells. There may be plenty of B cells in the blood, but they may not be as effective at producing antibodies in a high-fat environment — particularly a high-polyunsaturated-fat environment.

It's interesting to note that B cells usually get their marching orders from macrophages and T cells before they start producing antibodies. Possibly a high-fat diet suppresses the macrophage and T cell functions first, which in turn prevents these cells from sending out messenger chemicals (cytokines) to activate the B cells.

This would be similar to one way that HIV undermines the immune system: the disease destroys the CD4 cells, which essentially neutralizes the command centers of the immune system, and thus prevents B cells, killer T cells, and other immune defenses from being mobilized against an invader.

Arthritis, Fat, and Immunity

Fish Oils

Fish oils inhibit the production of interleukin-1 (IL-1), tumor necrosis factor, and prostaglandins, all of which cause inflammation. Recognizing fish oil's talent for inhibiting cytokines and inflammation, researchers speculated that fish oils could be used to suppress the immune response in people with autoimmune diseases, such as arthritis. And indeed, eighteen grams of fish oil per day for ten weeks caused a significant drop in symptoms, along with a decrease in the production of the cytokines IL-1 and tumor necrosis factor. The drop in cytokine production was greater than 60 percent.

In one study, as little as 2.6 grams of fish oil per day reduced arthritis symptoms, such as joint swelling, morning stiffness, and pain. Fish oil proved more effective than three to six grams of olive oil. These improvements, which took place over the twelve-week study period, paralleled reductions in blood levels of the proinflammatory cytokines (such as IL-1) and prostaglandins. In another report, seven hundred grams of fish per week (which amounts to four six-ounce servings of fish per week) had similar effects on cytokine levels and arthritis symptoms, as did 7.5 grams per day of fish oil.

Fish oil may not be the only arthritis-reducing source of omega-3 polyunsaturated fats. One study showed that black currant oil, which is rich in omega-6 fatty acids, had an effect similar to that of fish oils on subjects with rheumatoid arthritis. The levels of inflammation-promoting cytokines IL-1, IL-6, and tumor necrosis factor, as well as prostaglandin production by macrophages, decreased. Consumption of the oil also led to less morning stiffness.

Fish oils at twelve grams per day also seemed to slow the progression on another autoimmune disease called IgA nephropathy. In this disease, IgA antibody deposits in the kidney interfere with kidney function and can cause renal failure. Patients who had protein in their urine were helped by the fish oils.

Over the past twenty years, fat consumption in the United States has dropped from about 40 percent to 35 percent of the diet in terms of calories. We recommend an additional drop to 20 or 25 percent. Why not go still lower? There is epidemiological evidence suggesting that when fat consumption drops to 10 percent of total diet, an increased risk of strokes and death from ruptured blood vessels in the brain ensues. As with many other nutrients, we have to find the right balance.

References

De Logeril, M., S. Renaud, N. Mamelle, P. Salen, J. Martin, I. Monjaud, J. Guidollet, P. Touboul, and J. Celaye. "Mediterranean Alpha-Linolenic Acid–Rich Diet in Secondary Prevention of Coronary Artery Heart Disease." *Lancet* 343 (June 11, 1994): 1454–59.

Endres, S., S. Meydani, R. Ghorbani, R. Schindler, and C. Dinarello. "Dietary Supplementation with n-3 Fatty Acids Suppresses Inter-leukin-2 Production and Mononuclear Cell Proliferation." *Journal of Leukocyte Biology* 54 (December 1993): 599–603.

Fernandes, G. "Dietary Lipids and Risk of Autoimmune Disease." *Clinical Immunology and Immunopathology* 72 (August 1994): 193–97.

Geusens, P., C. Wouters, J. Nijs, Y. Jiang, and J. Dequeker. "Long-Term Effect of Omega-3 Fatty Acid Supplementation in Active Rheumatoid Arthritis: A 12-Month, Double-Blind, Controlled Study." *Arthritis and Rheumatism* 37 (June 1994): 824–29.

Herbert, J., J. Barone, M. Reddy, and J. Backlund. "Natural Killer Cell Activity in a Longitudinal Dietary Fat Intervention Trial." *Clinical Immunology and Immunopathology* 54 (January 1990): 103–16.

Jain, M., A. Miller, and T. To. "Premorbid Diet and the Prognosis of Women with Breast Cancer." *Journal of the National Cancer Institute* 86 (November 1, 1994): 1390–97.

Kelley, D., R. Dougherty, L. Branch, P. Taylor, and J. Iacono. "Concentration of Dietary n-6 Polyunsaturated Fatty Acids and the Human Immune Status." *Clinical Immunology and Immunopathology* 62 (February 1992): 240–44.

Kjeldsen-Kragh, J., M. Haugen, C. Borchgrevink, E. Laerum, M. Eek, P. Mowinkel, K. Hovi, and O. Forre. "Controlled Trial of Fasting and One-Year Vegetarian Diet in Rheumatoid Arthritis." *Lancet* 338 (October 12, 1991): 889–902.

Meydani, S., A. Lichtenstein, S. Cornwall, M. Meydani, B. Goldin, H. Rasmussen, C. Dinarello, and E. Schaefer. "Immunologic Effects of National Cholesterol Education Panel Step-2 Diets with and without Fish-Derived n-3 Fatty Acid Enrichment." *Journal of Clinical Investigations* 92 (July 1993): 105–13.

Ross, R. "The Pathogenesis of Atherosclerosis: A Perspective for the 1990s." *Nature* 362 (April 29, 1993): 801–9.

Watson, J., M. Byars, P. McGill, and A. Kelman. "Cytokine and Prostaglandin Production by Monocytes of Volunteers and Rheumatoid Arthritis Patients Treated with Dietary Supplements of Black Currant Seed Oil." *British Journal of Rheumatology* 32 (December 1993): 1055–58.

Willet, W. "Diet and Health: What Should We Eat?" *Science* 264 (April 22, 1994): 532–37.

CHAPTER NINETEEN

Medicinal Herbs, Spices, Cancer-Fighting Foods, and the Science

A NUMBER OF FOODS and medicinal plant derivatives have been examined for their immunity-boosting effects. Some have been used in folk medicine to heal immunity-related diseases such as infections and cancer; they have more recently been evaluated scientifically both to examine their efficacy and to understand how they work. Massive screening efforts are under way in hope of finding new wonder drugs based on natural products. The efforts are largely focused on plants used in folk medicine around the world. In this chapter, evidence is given to show the efficacy of some of these plant products.

Lentinan

Lentinan is a polysaccharide that comes from shiitake mushrooms, which is of the genus *Lentinula*. Recent research has shown that lentinan boosts a number of immune system activities. It can increase the killing of tumor cells by macrophages and natural killer cells in laboratory tests and has stimulated the macrophages of three out of five healthy volunteers injected with two milligrams of lentinan to produce the cytokine interleukin-6 (IL-6), which activates killing by macrophages. Lentinan is active in vitro at concentrations of twenty-five to one hundred nanograms per milliliter, a level manifested in patients' blood after lentinan treatment. Treated cancer patients also show an increase in natural killer cell and lymphokine-activated killer activity. These killer cells act like super natural killer cells and can destroy many types of cancer cells. In animal models, the mushroom extract boosts the ability of IL-2 to prevent the spread of cancer throughout the body.

In addition to its anticancer activity, lentinan's protective activity against infections is being confirmed by research. It increased levels of IL-6 in the lungs of mice and saved them from being killed by a potentially lethal respiratory infection with influenza virus. Lentinan also stimulates production of acute phase reactants and elevates levels of at least one of the complement byproducts, all of which help the body fight infections.

Garlic

Garlic is another food that has been promoted for its anti-infectious and anticancer properties. It has been used for many centuries in Chinese medicine. Research by and large supports its reputation. Epidemiological research shows an association of high garlic consumption and lower rates of gastric cancer in Italian and Chinese populations. Garlic (*Allium sativum*), wild garlic *(Allium ursinum),* and to a lesser extent, onions *(Allium cepa)* contain a family of thiol compounds that have been tested in the laboratory. Thiol compounds tend to have antioxidant activity. These compounds include allicin, ajoene, s-allylmercaptocysteine, and allyl alcohol. Garlic extracts boost a number of immune activities that could be related to controlling cancer. They stimulate T cell proliferation and enhance natural killer cell cytotoxic activity. They also enhance display of receptors for the cytokine IL-2 and enhance proliferation driven by IL-2. The activity of a garlic extract could be reversed with an antibody to IL-2, suggesting that the effect of garlic is to increase IL-2 levels. In another set of experiments, garlic extracts were shown to increase the oxidative burst of macrophages — that is, the production of oxygen-containing compounds that can kill infectious agents.

Garlic may also have anticancer effects that are independent of the immune system. Garlic extracts decrease the development of cancer after exposure to a number of oxidative mutagens such as radiation. The extracts were shown to lessen the oxidation of lipids by peroxides. These antioxidant properties could also help prevent heart disease.

In addition, evidence reveals an anti-infectious role for garlic compounds, independent of their immunity-boosting effects. Garlic compounds demonstrate both antibacterial and antiviral activity. One study showed that garlic extracts inhibited herpes simplex virus types 1 and 2, rhinovirus, vaccinia virus, and parainfluenza virus in the laboratory. Garlic compounds also inhibit the formation of thrombi by inhibiting platelet aggregation. They apparently block adhesion through integrins on the platelet surface. This might reduce the risk of strokes and cardiovascular disease.

Licorice

A less touted food that has been studied because of its immunity-building properties is licorice. A polysaccharide extract called glycyrrhizin, which is extracted from licorice root, has been used clinically and is said to have anti-inflammatory, antitumor, and antiviral activity. It stimulates enhanced display of IL-2 receptors and IL-2 production when added to cells in laboratory tests at two hundred micrograms per milliliter. It also stimulates phagocytosis by macrophages. In addition to glycyrrhizin, licorice root can contain ten different bioflavonoids. Their composition and quantity varies from species to species and even within the same species, depending on the place where it is grown.

Medicinal Plants

Echinacea

Echinacea is popularly recognized as an immunity-boosting herb. Its reputation is backed up by several studies showing immunity-modulating effects of water or ethanol extracts. It has been consistently shown to increase the ability of macrophages and granulocytes to phagocytize particles when added in laboratory experiments or when fed to animals or people. Polysaccharide extracts from echinacea could increase production of the inflammatory cytokines IL-1, IL-6, and tumor necrosis factor by macrophages. As a result of this activation, animals were protected against infections by several organisms that are best handled by phagocytes, including yeast infections. In spite of this apparent stimulatory activity, when applied directly to the skin an extract obtained from the root prevented an irritant from causing swelling and redness; that is, under these conditions it was anti-inflammatory.

The herb can induce opposite effects, depending on the way it is given. A moderate dose of extract, followed by a week without extract, stimulated lymphocyte multiplication and reaction to a skin test, whereas daily doses of a greater amount suppressed both reactions. This makes it tricky to calibrate dosages to produce desired effects but suggests that continued use is less effective than occasional use.

Mistletoe

A polysaccharide extracted from mistletoe *(Viscum album)* is being used in clinical trials in Germany as an antitumor agent. It stimulates the antitumor activity of macrophages, increasing the production of the cytokine tumor necrosis factor. It also inhibits the release of reactive oxygen compounds from granulocytes without weakening their overall ability to kill microorganisms. But one has to be careful, as mistletoe itself is poisonous and can cause miscarriages, convulsion, shock, and cardiac arrest.

Miscellaneous Medicinal Plants

Many other plant extracts with reputed health-promoting effects have been tested recently and shown to increase immunity. These include *Chamomilla recutita, Calendula officinalis, Ginkgo biloba, Tamarindus indica, Plantago asiatica, Larix occidentalis, Cassia garrettiana, Cnidium officinale, Tinospora malabarica, Osbeckia octandra, Melothria maderaspatana, Phyllanthus debelis,* and *Andrographis paniculata,* as well as several traditional herbal compositions.

For instance, treatment of mice with the Japanese herbal medicine sho-seiryu-to increased IgA antibody levels and increased resistance to infection with influenza virus. Mice were treated two times per day, starting on the day before infection and continuing for four days. In the same experiment, the pharmaceutical medicine Kakkon-to had no effect. A derivative of the bark of *Phellodendron amurense* was found to be the most potent agent within the Chinese traditional medicine *wen-qing-yin* for suppressing cell-mediated hypersensitivity reactions in mice. The herbal remedy *kanzo-bushi-to* inhibits the production of the cytokine interleukin-4 following burns and relieves burn-associated immunosuppression in mice. Natural killer cell activity increased in mice given *xiao-chai-hu-tang,* which might explain its efficacy for patients with chronic viral hepatitis. It also enhances production of the antibody IgA.

References

Aruna, K., and V. Sivaramakrishnan. "Anticarcinogenic Effects of Some Indian Plant Products." *Food and Chemical Toxicology* 30 (1992): 953–56.

Chan, M. "Inhibition of Tumor Necrosis Factor by Curcumin, a Phytochemical." *Biochemical Pharmacology* 49 (1995): 1551–56.

Chihara, G. "Recent Progress in Immunopharmacology and Therapeutic Effects of Polysaccharides." *Developments in Biological Standardization* 77 (1992): 191.

Chu, D., W. Wong, and G. Mavligit. "Immunotherapy with Chinese Medicinal Herbs. I. Immune Restoration of Local Xenogenic Graft-Versus-Host Reaction in Cancer Patients by Fractionated *Astragulus membranaceus* in Vitro." *Journal of Clinical and Laboratory Immunology* 25 (1988): 119–23.

Dorant, E., P. van den Brandt, R. Goldbohm, R. Hermus, and F. Sturmans. "Garlic and Its Significance for the Prevention of Cancer in Humans: A Critical Review." *British Journal of Cancer* 67 (March 1993): 424–29.

Haak-Frenscho, M., K. Kino, T. Sone, and P. Jardieu. "*Ling zhi-8:* A Novel T Cell Mitogen Induces Cytokine Production and Upregulation of ICAM-1 Expression." *Cellular Immunology* 150 (August 1993): 101–13.

Inamori, Y., M. Ogawa, H. Tsujibo, K. Baba, M. Kozawawa, and H. Nakamura. "Inhibitory Effects of 3,3',4,5'-Tetrahydroxystilbene and 3,3',4,5'–Tetrahydroxydibenzyl, the Constituents of *Cassia garrettiana* on Antigen-Induced Histamine Release in Vitro." *Pharmaceutical Bulletin* 39 (1991): 3353–54.

Kaneko, M., T. Kawakita, Y. Tauchi, Y. Saito, A. Suzuki, and K. Nomoto. "Augmentation of NK Activity After Oral Administration of a Traditional Chinese Medicine, *xiao-chai-hu-tang (shosaiko-to)*." *Immunopharmacology and Immunotoxicology* 16 (1994): 41–53.

Marwick, C. "Growing Use of Medicinal Botanicals Forces Assessment by Drug Regulators." *Journal of the American Medical Association* 273 (February 1995): 607–9.

Masuda, T., and A. Jitoe. "Antioxidative and Anti-Inflammatory Compounds from Tropical Gingers." *Journal of Agricultural Food Chemistry* 42 (September 1994): 1850–56.

Nair, S., M. Salomi, C. Varghese, B. Panikkar, and K. Panikkar. "Effect of Saffron on Thymocyte Proliferation, Intracellular Glutathione Levels, and Its Antitumor Activity." *Biofactors* 4 (December 1992): 51–54.

Pool, R. "Wrestling Anticancer Secrets from Garlic and Soy Sauce." *Science* 257 (September 4, 1992): 1348–49.

Roesler, J., A. Emmendorffer, C. Steinmuller, B. Luettig, J. Wagner, and M. Lohmnann-Matthes. "Application of Purified Polysaccharides from Cell Cultures of the Plant *Echinacea purpurea* to Test Subjects Mediate Activation of the Phagocyte System." *International Journal of Immunopharmacology* 13 (July 1991): 931–41.

Scaglione, R., F. Ferrara, S. Dugnani, M. Falchi, G. Santoro, and F. Fraschini. "Immunomodulatory Effects of Two Extracts of *Panax ginseng C. A. Meyer.*" *Drugs Under Experimental and Clinical Research* 16 (October 1990): 537–42.

Serafini, M., A. Ghiselli, and A. Ferro-Luzzi. "Red Wine, Tea, and Antioxidants." *Lancet* 344 (August 27, 1994): 626.

Suzuki, M., F. Takatsuki, Y. Maeda, J. Hamuro, and G. Chihara. "Antitumor and Immunological Activity of Lentinan in Comparison with LPS." *International Journal of Pharmacology* 16 (May–June 1994): 463–68.

't Hart, L., P. Nibbering, M. van den Barselaar, H. van Dijk, A. van den Berg, and R. Labadie. "Effects of Low Molecular Constituents from *Aloe vera* Gel on Oxidative Metabolism and Cytotoxic and Bactericidal Activities of Human Neutrophils." *International Journal of Immunopharmacology* 12 (December 1990): 427–34.

Tomoda, M., K. Takada, N. Shimizu, R. Gonda, and N. Ohara. "Reticuloendothelial System–Potentiating and Alkaline Phosphatase–Inducing Activities of Plantago-Mucilage A, the Main Mucilage from the Seed of *Plantago asiatica* and Its Five Modification Products." *Chemical and Pharmaceutical Bulletin* 39 (1991): 2068–71.

Weber, N., D. Andersen, J. North, B. Murray, L. Lawson, and B. Hughes. "In Vitro Virucidal Effects of *Allium sativum* (Garlic) Extract and Compounds." *Planta Medica* 58 (October 1992): 417–23.

Zhang, Y., K. Isobe, F. Nagase, T. Lwin, M. Kato, M. Hamaguchi, T. Yokochi, and I. Nakashima. "Glycyrrhizin as a Promoter of the Late Signal Transduction for Interleukin-2 Production by Splenic Lymphocytes." *Immunology* 79 (August 1993): 528–34.

CHAPTER TWENTY

Exercise and the Science

A s we exercise, our body produces stress hormones such as cortisol, adrenaline (epinephrine), and beta-endorphin. The amount and types of hormones produced vary with the type of exercise and its degree of difficulty. Exercise also oxygenates the blood, causing an oxidative stress associated with a brief decrease in glutathione, the blood's major antioxidant. Prolonged exercise can also lower levels of certain blood amino acids such as glutamine. Normally, muscle tissue makes a substantial amount of glutamine, which is an important energy source for cells of the immune system. During strenuous exercise, the amount of glutamine in the blood decreases. One theory holds that this energy starvation also contributes to the decrease of immunity brought on by heavy exercise. This theory is supported by a study that showed that giving glutamine to trained athletes helps them maintain a healthy immune response.

All of these factors can have an impact on immune system function. The effect of exercise on the system seems to depend strongly on the degree of exertion rather than the length of time spent.

The degree of physical exertion during exercise is rated using a measure called percent VO_2 max. It reflects the effort being exerted relative to a person's own maximum capacity. When this is done, the effects of exercise are fairly uniform across subjects;

that is, if you and I both exercise to 50 percent of our abilities, our immune systems would respond similarly even if I had to bicycle twice as vigorously to reach that state.

Another characteristic of exercise-induced immune system changes is that they tend to be short-lived. Most changes return to normal within fifteen minutes to two hours, although some last a day or more.

In general, the number of all major classes of white blood cells — granulocytes, monocytes, and lymphocytes — increases during exercise. Within the lymphocytes, CD8 cells are consistently reported to increase; some studies report an increase in CD4 cells, the helper cells, whereas others report a decrease. However, because CD8 cells, the suppressor or cytotoxic cells, increase more than CD4 cells, the CD4-CD8 ratio is consistently reported to decrease. Natural killer cells also increase. The granulocyte counts quickly return to preexercise levels. The monocytes return to baseline levels somewhat more slowly. Lymphocyte counts tend to drop below baseline levels an hour or so after exercising. The larger number of circulating cells arise from a redistribution of the cells within the body. The white blood cells leave resting places elsewhere in the body and enter the circulation.

Natural killer cell activity has been shown to increase during exercise in numerous studies. Again the effect is short-lived; the activity returns to normal or slightly below normal levels an hour or so after exercising. The increase in natural killer cell activity can be blocked by the drug naloxone, which blocks the effects of beta-endorphin. This suggests that the exercise caused an increase in beta-endorphin levels, which in turn caused an increase in natural killer activity. The decrease below baseline appeared to be due, in part, to the production of prostaglandins.

Macrophages also show signs of activation after exercise. Their ability to phagocytize and produce prostaglandin E and neopterin increases. Neopterin is a metabolite produced when macrophages are activated. There is also increased production of several cytokines, including interleukin-1 (IL-1) and interleukin-6 (IL-6).

Certain granulocyte activities are also enhanced. These include phagocytosis and chemotaxis — that is, the granulocytes' ability to find areas where they may be needed to gobble up invaders.

The ability of lymphocytes to multiply in response to a challenge is suppressed after exercise. Numerous studies report that responses to the mitogens conA, PHA, and PWM are all reduced. ConA and PHA stimulate T cells to divide, whereas PWM mostly stimulates B cells to divide. Again, the effect is usually short-lived, and the system returns to normal within an hour or two. The ability to make IL-2 is also reported to be reduced. The change in responsiveness is due in part to the relative decrease in CD4 cells. The number of B cells making antibodies (IgG, IgA, and IgM) also decreases. However, this effect seems to be secondary to a lack of help for the B cells. For instance, the ability of B cells to make antibodies to the Epstein-Barr virus is unusual in that in this case the B cells don't need help from T cells. This response to the virus does not change after exercise.

Nonetheless, there are also some signs of lymphocyte activation in vivo at least after prolonged exercise, as plasma levels of circulating IL-2 receptors, tumor necrosis factor receptors, the adhesion molecule ICAM-1 (intercellular adhesion molecule), and soluble CD8 increased in one study of runners after a five-hour alpine run.

Some studies have compared the immune systems of trained athletes to those of a control population. The levels of antibodies in blood and saliva, as well as the lymphocyte counts and proportion of T cells, were lower in the athletes. Natural killer cell activity was higher in the athletes. One study showed that glutamine could prevent the negative changes of immune function in trained athletes, presumably by countering the oxidative effects of exercise. A well-known connection exists between overtraining in athletes and an increased susceptibility to infections. This suggests that the net effect of consistent strenuous exercise is an impairment of an immune response to infections. A recent study showed that levels of IgA in the saliva dropped when runners ran on a treadmill on three successive days for ninety minutes at 75 percent VO_2. There was no decrease after just one session. This suggests that prolonged, repeated, high-intensity exercise has a cumulatively negative effect. Lower IgA levels would be expected to increase the risk of upper respiratory infections, as IgA is important in preventing bacteria and viruses from entering the body at mucosal surfaces.

The evidence suggests that only excessive levels of training are immunosuppressive. In a study of elderly women, those who were athletes had the lowest frequency of upper respiratory infections such as colds; those women who undertook a program of calisthenics had the greatest frequency of infections, and those who were in a walking program registered between the other two groups. Possibly the calisthenics were a greater exertion for the untrained women than the exercise for the conditioned women athletes. These results emphasize that the effects of exercise depend on the degree of exertion relative to a person's level of conditioning.

Cancer and Exercise

In general, a lower risk of cancer exists for people who exercise. A recent study showed that exercise reduced the risk of breast cancer in Caucasian women forty years old or younger, particularly those who had children. The researchers calculated the average exercise level from onset of menstruation to one year prior to the diagnosis of cancer. Those who exercised an average of at least forty-eight minutes per week were less likely to have developed cancer than those who exercised less or not at all. The greatest protection was seen in those who exercised the most, more than 3.8 hours per week. Their relative risk of developing breast cancer was 0.42 compared to those who didn't exercise. This analysis took into account the various other factors known to influence the development of breast cancer, such as age at first full-term pregnancy. It concluded that the decrease in ovarian hormones associated with exercise was protective.

Even moderate exercise may create problems for certain groups of people. Sedentary people over the age of fifty or those with diabetes, arthritis, obesity, circulatory problems, or emphysema, asthma, or other lung disorders should consult a doctor before starting an exercise program.

Aside from potential immunity-boosting effects, moderate exercise helps people sleep more easily, improves circulation, increases feelings of energy, and decreases feelings of fatigue, even in those with chronic fatigue syndrome.

References

Bernstein, L., B. Henderson, R. Hanisch, J. Sullivan-Halley, and R. Ross. "Physical Exercise and Reduced Risk of Breast Cancer in Young Women." *Journal of the National Cancer Institute* 86 (September 21, 1994): 1403–7.

Blair, S., H. Kohl, C. Barlow, R. Paffenbarger, L. Gibbons, and C. Macera. "Changes in Physical Fitness and All-Cause Mortality: A Prospective Study of Healthy and Unhealthy Men." *Journal of the American Medical Association* 273 (April 12, 1995): 1093–98.

Brenner, I., P. Shek, and R. Shepard. "Infection in Athletes." *Sports Medicine* 17 (1994): 86–107.

Hoffman-Goetz, L., and B. Klarlund Pedersen. "Exercise and the Immune System: A Model of the Stress Response?" *Immunology Today* 15 (August 1994): 382–87.

Nehlsen-Cannarella, S., D. Nieman, A. Balk-Lamberston, P. Markoff, D. Chritton, G. Gusewitch, and J. Lee. "The Effects of Moderate Exercise Training on Immune Response." *Medicine and Science in Sports and Exercise* 23 (January 1991): 64–70.

Nieman, D., D. Henson, G. Gusewitch, B. Warren, R. Dotson, D. Butterworth, and S. Nehlsen-Cannarella. "Physical Activity and Immune Function in Elderly Women." *Medicine and Science in Sports and Exercise* 25 (July 1993): 823–31.

Ortega, E., C. Barriga, and M. de la Fuente. "Study of the Phagocytic Process in Neutrophils from Elite Sportswomen." *European Journal of Applied Physiology and Occupational Physiology* 66 (January 1993): 37–42.

Peters, E., J. Goetzsche, B. Grobbelaar, and T. Noakes. "Vitamin C Supplementation Reduces the Incidence of Postrace Symptoms of Upper-Respiratory-Tract Infection in Ultramarathon Runners." *American Journal of Clinical Nutrition* 57 (February 1993): 170–74.

Shephard, R., T. Verde, S. Thomas, and P. Shek. "Physical Activity and the Immune System." *Canadian Journal of Sport Sciences* 16 (September 1991): 169–85.

CHAPTER TWENTY-ONE

Mind, Body, and the Science

I N THINKING ABOUT THE effects of stress on immune function and health, one has to make a distinction between *distress* and what is called *eustress* — a good form of stress. Examples of stressful situations include too much work and too little time, parachuting from an airplane, and so on. Each of these can be seen as an exciting challenge, in which case they would cause eustress; they could also be viewed as threatening or frustrating, in which case they would cause distress. In the most general terms, distress is thought to impair the function of lymphocytes, whereas eustress either enhances immunity or has no effect on it. The key to handling stress is our reaction to it.

In a recent review, Dr. Bruce McEwen of the Rockefeller Institute discussed the nature of stress, its physiological consequences, and its relationship to disease. He emphasized the differences in individual responses to stress and its interaction with the biosocial setting. He compared the difference in probable response to the same work situation, for example, being asked to see the boss, for a secure employee and for one who feels in danger of losing his or her job. At another level, he discussed how stress affects both the cardiovascular and immune systems, and how the outcome of stress is further influenced by other lifestyle factors. For instance, monkeys under social stress have increased atherosclerosis, which becomes a much more serious health threat if they are also on a high-fat diet. Thus, the effect of stress depends upon a number of factors, some or all of which we can influence. Aside from its effects on the immune system, stress is thought to contribute to the development of heart disease, asthma, ulcers, inflammatory bowel syndrome, diabetes, migraine headaches, and premenstrual syndrome.

Neuroendocrine Mediators

There is an overlap between the hormones produced in response to stress that contribute to cardiovascular disease and those that cause immune dysfunction. In the face of stress, the body produces a variety of neurochemicals, both neurotransmitters and neurohormones. The most prominently studied have been cortisol and the catecholamines, epinephrine (adrenaline), and norepinephrine (noradrenaline). However, many other neurohormones, such as the endorphins and enkephalins (endogenous opiates), prolactin, and melatonin are also postulated to play a role. These agents generally share the ability to modulate signaling between the cell's surface receptors and its nucleus. In this way they can either amplify or interfere with the ability of immune cells to respond effectively to a challenge.

The levels of neurohormones are usually tightly regulated. High levels of cortisol, for instance, feed back to turn off further production of cortisol. This to some extent leads to a cyclical daily pattern in levels of cortisol and other stress hormones. The body also tries to adapt to stress by reducing the number of receptors on immune cells for a neurochemical that is present at high levels. In animal studies, repeated exposure to stress, such as electrical shocks, causes the animal to adapt to the stress, so that over time the shocks lose their immunosuppressive effect. However, in human studies, where stressors are more often interpersonal, the immunosuppressive effects of stress tend to persist, as is seen with caregivers of patients with Alzheimer's disease.

Several conditions are associated with abnormal levels of stress hormones or an abnormal hormonal response to stress. These include aging, which predisposes a person to hyperresponsiveness to stress; depression, in which cortisol levels are often high and normal feedback mechanisms don't work; and certain autoimmune disease models, in which it is thought that low levels of cortisol or its equivalent allow the immune system to become overreactive and thereby start attacking the body's own tissues.

Lymphocytes, monocytes, and granulocytes all have receptors for these neurochemicals. One of the more astounding developments in the field of psychoneuroimmunology has been the increasing evidence that the immune system and central nervous system share signaling molecules. Not only do lymphocytes respond to neurochemicals, but they can also produce many of them themselves. In addition, the brain has receptors for and responds to certain cytokines. Most recently, the brain has also been shown to be able to make cytokines such as interleukin-1. Thus the distinction between neurochemicals and cytokines has become blurred. This makes a certain amount of sense, since both the immune system and the nervous system share many of the same goals: they both react to our environment and commit their experiences to memory.

Consequences for the Immune System

A variety of immune system functions are influenced by stress. Dr. Tracey Herbert and Dr. Sheldon Cohen at Carnegie Mellon University in Pittsburgh recently combined the results of thirty-eight publications on the effects of stress on immunity in humans. The strongest and most consistent effects are decreases in the multiplication of lymphocytes in response to stimulation with the mitogens PHA and conA, and decreases in natural killer cell activity. (PHA and conA are plant-derived substances that stimulate the majority of T lymphocytes to divide.) In one study, changes in natural killer cell activity paralleled changes in norepinephrine. The production of cytokines such as interleukin-2 and gamma-interferon is also reported to decrease. However, interleukin-1 secretion has been reported to increase. Antibodies to herpes viruses tend to be elevated. Herpes viruses lurk in the body forever after the initial infection. They are generally dormant, but when the cells of the immune system are weakened, the virus becomes reactivated. The body responds by making antibodies to the virus. An increase in antibodies to herpes viruses is interpreted as suggesting that the T lymphocyte immunity responsible for controlling these viruses has been suppressed. A number of studies report that the CD4-CD8 ratio decreases, most often because the number of CD8 cells increases. The number of granulocytes in the blood also increases. Similar changes have been reported for people suffering from chronic stress.

The largest body of evidence for the effects of stress on immunity in everyday life has been produced by Ronald Glaser and Janice Kiecolt-Glaser at Ohio State University. They have studied medical students at exam time, recently divorced individuals, caregivers to sufferers of Alzheimer's disease, and married couples discussing their differences. The results are generally consistent across groups.

Neurochemicals such as prolactin, melatonin, and growth hormone stimulate immunity in laboratory experiments. Although more work needs to be done in this area, it seems likely that situations promoting the production of such neurochemicals would support a more effective immune system. This, at least in part, may be the way feelings of security, affection, or self-esteem protect us.

References

Stress

Ader, R., N. Cohen, and D. Felten. "Psychoneuroimmunology: Interactions Between the Nervous System and the Immune System." *Lancet* 345 (January 14, 1995): 99–102.

Alexander, C., H. Shandler, E. Langer, R. Newman, and J. Davies. "Transcendental Meditation, Mindfulness, and Longevity: An Experimental Study with the Elderly." *Journal of Personality and Social Psychology* 57 (1989): 950–64.

Benson, H. *The Relaxation Response.* New York: Morrow, 1975.

Cohen, S., D. Tyrrell, and A. Smith. "Psychological Stress and Susceptibility to the Common Cold." *New England Journal of Medicine* 325 (August 29, 1991): 606–12.

Dekaris, D., A. Sabioncello, R. Mazuran, S. Rabatic, I. Svoboda-Beusan, L. Racunica, and J. Tomaasic. "Multiple Changes of Immunologic Parameters in Prisoners of War: Assessments After Release from a Camp in Manjaca, Bosnia." *Journal of the American Medical Association* 270 (August 4, 1993): 595–99.

Fawzy, F., N. Fawzy, L. Arndt, and R. Pasnau. "Critical Review of Psychosocial Interventions in Cancer Care." *Archives of General Psychiatry* 52 (February 1995): 100–13.

Fernstrom, J. "Dietary Amino Acids and Brain Function." *Journal of the American Dietetic Association* 94 (January 1994): 71–77.

Groer, M., J. Mozingo, P. Droppleman, M. Davis, M. Jolly, M. Boynton, K. Davis, and S. Kay. "Measures of Salivary Secretory Immunoglobulin A and State of Anxiety After a Nursing Back Rub." *Applied Nursing Research* 7 (February 1994): 2–6.

Herbert, T., and S. Cohen. "Stress and Immunity in Humans: A Meta-analytic Review." *Psychosomatic Medicine* 55 (July–August 1993): 364–79.

Knapp, P., E. Levy, R. Giorgi, P. Black, and B. and T. Heeren. "Short-Term Immunological Effects of Induced Emotion." *Psychosomatic Medicine* 54 (March–April 1992): 133–48.

Lieberman, H., J. Wurtman, and M. Teicher. "Aging, Nutrient Choice,

Activity, and Behavioral Responses to Nutrients." *Annals of the New York Academy of Sciences* 561 (1989): 196–208.

McEwen, B. "Stress and the Individual: Mechanisms Leading to Disease." *Archives of Internal Medicine* 153 (September 27, 1993): 2093–101.

Moyers, B. D. *Healing and the Mind.* New York: Doubleday, 1993.

Ornish, D. *Stress, Diet, and Your Heart.* New York: Holt Rinehart & Winston, 1982.

Pennebaker, J., J. Kiecolt-Glaser, and R. Glaser. "Disclosure of Traumas and Immune Function: Health Implications for Psychotherapy." *Journal of Consulting and Clinical Psychology* 56 (April 1988): 239–45.

Sheridan, J., C. Dobbs, D. Brown, and B. Zwilling. "Psychoneuroimmunology: Stress Effects on Pathogenesis and Immunity During Infection." *Clinical Microbiology Reviews* 7 (April 1994): 200–12.

Sobrian, S., V. Vaughn, E. Bloch, and L. Burton. "Influence of Prenatal Maternal Stress on the Immunocompetence of the Offspring." *Pharmacology, Biochemistry and Behavior* 43 (October 1992): 537–47.

Zachariae, R., J. Kristensen, P. Hokland, J. Ellegaard, E. Metze, and M. Hokland. "Effect of Psychological Intervention in the Form of Relaxation and Guided Imagery on Cellular Immune Function in Normal Healthy Subjects." *Psychotherapy and Psychosomatics* 54 (January 1990): 32–39.

Mood and Attitude

Greer, S., T. Morris, K. Pettingale, and J. Haybittle. "Psychological Response to Breast Cancer and 15-Year Outcome." *Lancet* 335 (January 6, 1990): 49–50.

Irwin, M., M. Daniels, T. Smith, E. Bloom, and H. Weiner. "Impaired Natural Killer Cell Activity During Bereavement." *Brain, Behavior, and Immunity* 1 (March 1987): 98–104.

Laudenslager, M., S. Ryan, R. Drugan, R. Hyson, and S. Maier. "Coping and Immunosuppression: Inescapable but Not Escapable Shock Suppresses Lymphocyte Proliferation." *Science* 221 (August 5, 1983): 568–70.

Levy, E., D. Borrelli, S. Mirin, P. Salt, P. Knapp, C. Peirce, B. Fox, and P.

Black. "Biological Measures and Cellular Immunological Function in Depressed Psychiatric Inpatients." *Psychiatry Research* 36 (February 1991): 157–67.

Maes, M., S. Scharpe, H. Meltzer, E. Bosmans, E. Suy, J. Calabrese, and P. Cosyns. "Relationship Between Interleukin-6 Activity, Acute Phase Proteins, and Function of the Hypothalamic-Pituitary-Adrenal Axis in Severe Depression." *Psychiatry Research* 49 (October 1993): 11–27.

McGee, R., S. Williams, and M. Elwood. "Depression and the Development of Cancer: A Meta-Analysis." *Social Science and Medicine* 38 (January 1994): 187–92.

Peterson, C., S. Maier, and M. Seligman. *Learned Helplessness: A Theory for the Age of Personal Control.* New York: Oxford University Press, 1993.

Phillips, D., T. Ruth, and L. Wagner. "Psychology and Survival." *Lancet* 342 (November 6, 1993): 1142–45.

Selye, H. *The Stress of Life.* New York: McGraw-Hill, 1956.

Sieber, W., J. Rodin, L. Larson, S. Ortega, and N. Cummings. "Modulation of Human Natural Killer Cell Activity by Exposure to Uncontrollable Stress." *Brain, Behavior, and Immunity* 6 (June 1992): 141–56.

Relationships

Davis, M., J. Neuhaus, D. Moritz, and M. Segal. "Living Arrangements and Survival Among Middle-Aged and Older Adults in the NHANES I Epidemiologic Follow-up Study." *American Journal of Public Health* 82 (March 1992): 401–6.

Kiecolt-Glaser, J., J. Dura, C. Speicher, P. Trask, and R. Glaser. "Spousal Caregivers of Dementia Victims: Longitudinal Changes in Immunity and Health." *Psychosomatic Medicine* 53 (July–August 1991): 345–62.

Kiecolt-Glaser, J., L. Fisher, P. Ogrocki, J. Stout, C. Speicher, and R. Glaser. "Marital Quality, Marital Disruption, and Immune Function." *Psychosomatic Medicine* 49 (January–February 1987): 13–34.

Kiecolt-Glaser, J., S. Kennedy, S. Malkoff, L. Fisher, C. Speicher, and

R. Glaser. "Marital Discord and Immunity in Males." *Psychosomatic Medicine* 50 (May–June 1988): 213–29.

Kiecolt-Glaser, J., W. Malarkey, M. Chee, T. Newton, J. Cacioppo, H. Mao, and R. Glaser. "Negative Behavior During Marital Conflict Is Associated with Immunological Down-Regulation." *Psychosomatic Medicine* 55 (September–October 1993): 395–409.

Ruberman, W. "Psychosocial Influences on Mortality of Patients with Coronary Heart Disease." *Journal of the American Medical Association* 267 (January 22–29, 1992): 559–60.

Spiegel, D., J. Bloom, H. Kraemer, and E. Gottheil. "Effect of Psychosocial Intervention on Survival of Patients with Metastatic Breast Cancer." *Lancet* ii (December 16, 1989): 888–91.

CHAPTER TWENTY-TWO

Staying Out of Harm's Way:
The Science

A HOST OF FACTORS can harm the immune system. Among these are recreational drugs including alcohol, certain medications, pollution, and lack of sleep.

Alcohol

Alcohol is perhaps the best studied of these factors. There is little evidence that low levels (say, blood levels following one drink) of alcohol suppress immunity; however, high levels suppress a variety of immune system functions. In nonalcoholics, the effects of alcohol seem to be short-lived and return to normal as the alcohol is cleared from the body. Alcoholics show less lymphocyte multiplication in response to stimulation, whether or not they have developed liver disease. Even after years of abuse, however, the immune defects are at least partly reversible over a period of months, if a person stops drinking. Alcoholics are much more susceptible than the general public to infections, but this is difficult to attribute solely to alcohol because nutritional deficiencies, including low levels of zinc, are often present in alcoholics as well.

Most experiments either have looked for direct effects of alcohol in tests of human or animal immune cells exposed to alcohol outside the body, or have tested immune cells following several weeks of a diet that contains alcohol. Usually results using the two methods agree, suggesting that many of the effects of alcohol on immune cells are direct ones; that is, the effects are due to the alcohol itself rather than secondary changes in hormones or behaviors associated with alcohol use.

Lymphocytes, monocytic cells, and granulocytes are all affected by high doses of alcohol. Lymphocytes are less able to divide in response to mitogenic stimulation or to respond in skin-test experiments. In one experiment with rats that looked at gender differences in response to alcohol, levels of antibodies increased and mitogen responses decreased only in females, whereas CD4 lymphocyte counts went up only in males. Natural killer cell destruction of tumor cells was variably affected and, depending on the experimental setup, was suppressed, enhanced, or didn't change.

More important, macrophages from the lungs (alveolar macrophages) and the liver (Kupffer's cells) are both less able to produce superoxide radicals (which kill microorganisms) when exposed to alcohol. Macrophages are also less able to produce the cytokines tumor necrosis factor, interleukin-1 (IL-1), and granulocyte-macrophage colony-stimulating factor (an important factor for stimulating the bone marrow to produce more macrophages and granulocytes). They are also less able to provide help to T lymphocytes. Prostaglandin production is, however, increased. These changes leave heavy alcohol users less able to fight infections.

Several studies have also looked at combined effects of diet and alcohol. In one study, alcohol was more suppressive of Kupffer's cell IL-1 production in rats that were fed a diet high in unsaturated fat, compared to rats that were fed saturated fats. In the same study, only the rats on the diet with unsaturated fat and alcohol developed liver disease. Other studies have shown that nutritionally inadequate diets compound the effects of alcohol on immunity. The combined effect of alcohol and nicotine suppresses natural killer cell activity at levels that neither one alone could.

Children of women who drink large amounts of alcohol during pregnancy are at risk of developing fetal alcohol syndrome. These children have low lymphocyte multiplication responses and are at greater risk of infection throughout childhood. Several groups have been studying this phenomenon in animal models. Chronic exposure of pregnant females to alcohol results in male offspring whose lymphocyte responses to mitogen are impaired into adulthood. Studies show the T lymphocytes cannot utilize IL-2 effectively (this cytokine helps T lymphocytes divide). One study using monkeys found the lymphocytes from mothers fed alcohol during pregnancy were less able to multiply in response to the antigen that causes tetanus, and less able to make antibodies to this antigen when immunized with it. The offspring were also more susceptible to infection.

The effects in children seem to be a consequence of neuroendocrine changes caused by alcohol during gestation. The offspring themselves have abnormal neuroendocrine responses. In one recent experiment, Dr. Eva Redei at the University of Pennsylvania in Philadelphia showed that male offspring had abnormally high levels of messenger RNA for the pro-opiomelanocortin (POMC) molecule in the anterior pituitary gland. POMC codes for endogenous opioids, melanocyte-stimulating hormone, and the hormone that causes cortisol to be released. Data suggested that elevated levels of cortisol in the mother during pregnancy caused the abnormalities in the developing child. In human studies it takes at least three drinks to elevate cortisol levels. Other experiments have shown an abnormal fever response and an abnormal neuroendocrine response to interleukin-1.

Most immunosuppressive effects of alcohol occur when enough alcohol has been imbibed to render the drinker legally drunk. The dangers to health mainly come from heavy chronic drinking. Of particular concern is heavy use (greater than two drinks per day) of alcohol during pregnancy, because it affects the child's development and can cause long-lasting problems.

Psychoactive Recreational Drugs

Cocaine

A number of T cell functions are impaired by cocaine in animal models. These include killing by T cells and the production of the cytokines gamma-interferon, tumor necrosis factor, and the T cell growth factors IL-2 and IL-4. Regarding T cell multiplication, there is either no effect or stimulation at low doses and suppression at high doses. The effects on the immune system appear to be indirect, since adding cocaine directly to T cells in laboratory experiments either has no effect or sometimes an effect opposite to that seen in animals. The higher the dose of cocaine, the longer the body takes to recover from its effects, which last from one to several days.

Cocaine also suppresses a number of macrophage functions. It suppresses killing by macrophages, production of the cytokines IL-1 and tumor necrosis factor, phagocytosis, and nitric oxide production. The effects of cocaine on macrophages may be more direct; in laboratory experiments cocaine also inhibits the production of oxygen products by macrophages, which are lethal to microorganisms. Granulocyte chemotaxis, the ability of these cells to move toward a chemical signal, is also decreased. These factors leave cocaine users more susceptible to infections. People recently exposed to cocaine have fewer circulating CD4 T cells and more natural killer cells. These lymphocytes show more evidence of activation, but it is hard to know whether this is because cocaine activated them or because more infections stimulated them.

Heroin, Morphine, and Methadone

Lymphocytes from intravenous drug users tend to respond less well to mitogens, and these drug users have higher levels of IgG and IgM antibodies in their blood. The levels of CD4 cells are lower than in nonusers. As with alcohol, the effects of intravenous drugs can have long-lasting effects on immunity in the children of women who continue to use drugs during pregnancy. Lymphocytes of infants of intravenous drug abusers multiply less well when challenged and have lower CD4-CD8 ratios.

In animal models, morphine, the major metabolite of heroin, causes decreased superoxide production and decreased gamma-interferon, IL-1, and tumor necrosis factor production, as well as less killing by macrophages. Methadone also decreases superoxide production but does not weaken monocytic cytokine production. These abnormalities typically lead to greater susceptibility to infections.

Marijuana

Most studies of marijuana have examined the effect of its major psychoactive component, delta-tetrahydrocannabinol (DTHC). In animal studies, repeated exposure over a period of weeks suppresses natural killer cell destruction of tumor cells and interferon production. In laboratory experiments, DTHC at levels such as those found in the blood after a person had smoked marijuana increased interferon production, but interferon production was suppressed by higher levels of the drug. One study examined the effect of a nonpsychoactive component of marijuana, cannabidiol. It could suppress IL-1 and tumor necrosis factor production. Macrophage phagocytosis was suppressed by exposure to a physiological dose of DTHC. This suggests that macrophages and natural killer cells may be more sensitive than lymphocytes to the suppressive effects of marijuana. The net effects of marijuana use on immunity could make heavy users more susceptible to infections and possibly cancer.

Miscellaneous Psychoactive Recreational Drugs

Other recreational drugs are less well studied, but scattered reports suggest that LSD, PCP, amphetamines, and nitrite inhalants can all be immunosuppressive. The hallucinogen LSD suppresses B cell multiplication and the production of the cytokines IL-2, IL-4, and IL-6 in laboratory experiments when added in biologically reasonable amounts. Natural killer cell activity is suppressed by high levels and enhanced by low amounts.

PCP suppresses IL-2 production at moderate levels and cytotoxic T cell activity at high concentrations. It can also suppress B and T lymphocyte multiplication. Macrophage production of cytokines is not suppressed.

Amphetamine action depended on the form of the drug. Amphetamine itself suppressed IL-2 but not IL-4 production and B cell multiplication in laboratory experiments; the synthetic amphetamine cathinone stimulated IL-2 cell production, B cell multiplication, and cytotoxic T cell killing. Methamphetamine stimulated natural killer cell activity.

Nitrite inhalants lowered the number of T cells in the blood of volunteers and natural killer cell activity but had no effect on lymphocyte multiplication. In animal studies, exposure reduced the ability to produce antibodies and antigen-presenting cell activity by macrophages.

Pharmaceutical Medications

Relatively few medications have been studied for their effect on the immune system. As would be expected from the interaction of the brain and the immune system, many of the drugs used to treat depression and anxiety seem to affect immunity.

These include drugs that modulate neurotransmitters in the brain. Some of these drugs can prevent stress-induced immuno-suppression and infections in animal models. These include al-prazolam, diazepam, metipranolol, and terguride. However, in laboratory experiments diazepam inhibited phagocytic function and antibody synthesis. Lithium carbonate has immunostimula-tory properties.

A number of drugs used as anesthetics are immunosuppres-sive and may contribute to the immunosuppression seen after surgery. Phenobarbital, ketamine/xylazine, and chloral hydrate cause immunosuppression of antibody production that lasts for at least a week in an animal model. Halothane and meth-oxyflurane had no effect on antibody production. Halothane did, however, suppress natural killer cell destruction of tumor cells, as did Avertin, isoflurane, ether, and ketamine/xylazine.

Several antibiotics have been found to suppress cell-mediated immunity. These include prodigiosin 25-C, mezlocillin, rifam-picin, and doxycycline. Roxithromycin and trimethoprim also in-hibited superoxide generation by the granulocytes. Not all antibi-otics weakened T cell immunity. Drugs that had no effect on cell-mediated immunity in one study include vancomycin, teico-planin, penicillin G, piperacillin, cefamandole, cefotaxime, gen-tamicin, amikacin, streptomycin, and clindamycin. Clindamycin, however, moderately suppressed the ability of granulocytes to make the toxic oxygen-containing products after gobbling up microorganisms. At least one antibiotic studied so far is immu-nostimulatory. Ciprofloxacin stimulates cytokine production of IL-1, IL-2, and gamma-interferon, which typically boost T cell activity.

Caffeine

Caffeine is a methylxanthine that changes cellular levels of cAMP, a message the cell uses to signal the nucleus to make new proteins. Caffeine has inhibited the multiplication of B and T cells in laboratory experiments and can also reduce T cell cytokine production.

Cigarettes

Although lymphocyte multiplication and natural killer cell activity have been reported to be lower in smokers, in only some studies, alveolar macrophages (those from the lungs) are consistently reported to be abnormal in smokers. They produce fewer superoxide radicals, are less able to eat up microorganisms, and express less class II MHC on their surfaces. They are more susceptible to herpes simplex infection and less able to kill internalized bacteria. IL-1 production, on the other hand, is increased. Granulocytes are also less able to phagocytize. This combination would explain why smokers are more prone to respiratory infections. Smokers also respond less well to vaccination than do nonsmokers, in spite of having generally elevated levels of antibodies. The combination of nicotine and alcohol suppresses immune response in ways that neither one could do on its own. Also, an antigen purified from tobacco is shown to stimulate production of the cytokines IL-1 and IL-6, which stimulate inflammation, and IgE, the antibody involved in allergic reactions.

Other changes associated with smoking are an elevation in the number of T lymphocytes in the blood, particularly CD4 cells, and a decrease in plasma levels of vitamin C and beta-carotene.

Fortunately, several studies show that the immune system begins to return to normal within a few months after smoking cessation.

Environmental Toxins

The most widely studied class of toxins is the aromatic hydrocarbons. A marked relation exists between the carcinogenic potential of these compounds and their immunosuppressive effects. These compounds, which include herbicides such as dioxin and benzopyrene, are found in automobile exhaust and smoke from industrial and municipal plants. These compounds can depress cell-mediated immunity (T cell and macrophage function) and interfere with the production of both B and T cells; they induce B cells to self-destruct.

These compounds bind to a receptor inside the cell that has similarities to the steroid receptor. Once bound, the aromatic hydrocarbon can be transported to the nucleus, where it can cause mutations in the cell's DNA. Binding can be inhibited by certain bioflavonoids, compounds which occur in tea and a variety of vegetables. Because the bioflavonoids compete for the same receptor and keep it occupied, they prevent these environmental toxins from getting to the nucleus and causing damage. Unfortunately, there are "good" bioflavonoids and "bad" ones. The good ones block toxins, but the bad ones mimic the activity of the toxins.

Certain heavy metals also suppress immune function. In animal models, both aluminum and mercury salts restrict the ability of T lymphocytes to produce cytokines, particularly gamma-interferon. Mercury salts induce autoimmune disease in certain strains of mice, depending on their genetically determined MHC type. Occupational exposure to lead in a group of firearm instructors decreased the ability of their T lymphocytes to multiply. B lymphocyte function was unaffected. It was suggested that lead interfered with antigenic presentation because it binds strongly to the T cell receptor and MHC class II antigens. The firearm instructors also had fewer than normal CD4 lymphocytes.

Ultraviolet rays impair T cell cytokine production, and ultraviolet exposure in general stimulates suppressor cells. This suppression could contribute to the development of skin cancer that occurs with too much exposure to sunlight.

A number of the factors mentioned here are especially detrimental during pregnancy. Radiation and pesticide exposure during pregnancy can cause long-lasting immune system changes in infants and leave them more vulnerable to infections.

References

Criqui, M., and B. Ringel. "Does Diet of Alcohol Explain the French Paradox?" *Lancet* 344 (December 24–31, 1994): 1719–23.

Culver, K., A. Amman, J. Partridge, D. Wong, D. Wara, and M. Cowan. "Lymphocyte Abnormalities in Infants Born to Drug-Abusing Mothers." *Journal of Pediatrics* 111 (February 1987): 230–35.

Doric, N. M., M. Abram, and T. Rukavina. "Antimicrobial Activity and Immunological Side Effects of Different Antibiotics." *Folia Biologica* 39 (March 1993): 162–65.

Fischbein, A., P. Tsang, J. Luo, J. Roboz, J. Jiang, and J. Bekesi. "Phenotypic Aberrations of CD3+ and CD4+ Cells and Functional Impairment of Lymphocytes at Low-Level Occupational Exposure to Lead." *Clinical Immunology and Immunopathology* 66 (February 1993): 163–68.

Henningfield, J. "Nicotine Medications for Smoking Cessation." *New England Journal of Medicine* 333 (November 2, 1995): 1196–202.

Holsapple, M., and A. Munson. "Immunotoxicology of Abused Drugs." In *Immunotoxicology and Immunopharmacology,* edited by J. Dean et al. New York: Raven Press, 1985.

Irwin, M., T. Smith, and J. Gillin. "Electroencephalographic Sleep and Natural Killer Activity in Depressed Patients and Control Subjects." *Psychosomatic Medicine* 54 (January–February 1992): 10–21.

Ladics, G., T. Kawabata, and K. White. "Suppression of the in Vitro Humoral Immune Response of Mouse Splenocytes by 7, 12-dimethylbenz[a]anthracene Metabolites and Inhibition of Immunosuppression by α-naphthoflavone." *Toxicology and Applied Pharmacology* 110 (August 1991): 31–44.

Lefkowitz, S., A. Vaz, and D. Lefkowitz. "Cocaine Reduces Macrophage

Killing by Inhibiting Reactive Nitrogen Intermediates." *International Journal of Immunopharmacology* 15 (1993): 717–21.

Peterson, P., G. Gekker, C. Brummitt, P. Pentel, M. Bullock, M. Simpson, J. Hitt, and B. Sharp. "Suppression of Human Peripheral Blood Mononuclear Cell Function by Methadone and Morphine." *Journal of Infectious Diseases* 159 (March 1989): 480–87.

Redei, E., I. Halasz, L. Li, M. Prystowsky, and F. Aird. "Maternal Adrenalectomy Alters the Immune and Endocrine Functions of Fetal Alcohol-Exposed Male Offspring." *Endocrinology* 133 (August 1993): 452–60.

Szabo, G., B. Verma, and D. Catalano. "Selective Inhibition of Antigen-Specific T Lymphocyte Proliferation by Acute Ethanol Exposure: The Role of Impaired Monocyte Antigen Presentation Capacity and Mediator Production." *Journal of Leukocyte Biology* 54 (1993): 534–44.

Tappia, P., K. Troughton, S. Langley-Evans, and R. Grimble. "Cigarette Smoking Influences Cytokine Production and Antioxidant Defences." *Clinical Science* 88 (April 1995): 485–89.

Watson, R., P. Borgs, M. Witte, R. McCuskey, C. Lantz, M. Johnson, S. Mufti, and D. Earnest. "Alcohol, Immunomodulation, and Disease." *Alcohol and Alcoholism* 29 (March 1994): 131–39.

Watzl, B., P. Scuder, and R. Watson. "Marijuana Components Stimulate Human Peripheral Blood Mononuclear Cell Secretion of Interferon-Gamma and Suppress Interleukin-1 Alpha in Vitro." *International Journal of Immunopharmacology* 13 (1991): 1091–97.

Winter, A., E. Follett, J. Mcintrye, J. Stewart, and I. Symington. "Influence of Smoking on Immunological Responses to Hepatitis B Vaccine." *Vaccine* 12 (1994): 771–74.

Glossary

Adhesion molecule: a cell surface protein that helps cells stick to other cells or the materials in between cells.

Antibody: a circulating protein, produced by B lymphocytes, that can recognize an antigen and aid in its clearance (*antibody* and *immunoglobulin* mean the same thing).

Antigen: any molecule capable of being recognized by a B or T lymphocyte, thus potentially stimulating an immune response.

Basophil: a type of granulocyte involved in allergies.

B cell: a lymphocyte that has the potential to make antibodies. It uses antibody molecules on its surface to recognize antigen.

CD4: a protein characteristically present on the membrane of helper T lymphocytes. CD4 binds to class II MHC molecules on antigen-presenting cells.

CD8: a protein characteristically present on the surface of cytotoxic and suppressor T lymphocytes.

Cell-mediated immunity: refers to immunity that involves a T cell response.

Complement: a group of serum proteins that create byproducts involved in inflammation, phagocytosis, and cell destruction.

Cytokine: a small protein often produced by immune cells that communicates signals to stimulate or suppress the function of other immune and nonimmune cells. Cytokines are synonymous with interleukins and are also sometimes called lymphokines or monokines.

Cytotoxic T cell: a T cell that recognizes and kills other cells.

Granulocyte: the most abundant form of white blood cell. Granulocytes are phagocytic cells that contain toxic granules. The three types of granulocytes are neutrophils, eosinophils, and basophils. Granulocytes are also called polymorphonuclear cells.

Helper T cell: a class of T lymphocyte that is important in stimulating the function of other immune cells.

Humoral: referring to processes taking place in the plasma or other fluids of the body, usually implying an antibody-mediated immune response.

Hypersensitivity: an overly strong immune response that leads to tissue damage.

Immune complex: a complex of antigen and antibody.

Immunoglobulin: see *Antibody.*

Inflammation: the response to injury or infection involving increased blood flow and entry of white blood cells into the tissues, which results in swelling, redness, heat, and pain.

Innate immunity: immunity that is present without prior exposure to antigen.

Integrins: a class of adhesion molecules.

Interferon: a subclass of cytokines with antiviral properties.

Interleukin (IL): cytokines. Different types of interleukins follow.

IL-1: produced by macrophages; stimulates immune cells and also causes fever and other systemic reactions to infection.

IL-2: produced by T cells; acts as a growth factor for T cells and stimulates T cell activity.

IL-4: produced by certain helper T cells; stimulates antibody production and inhibits macrophage activation.

IL-10: produced by T cells that make IL-4; suppresses other T cells so that they stop making interferon.

IL-12: produced by natural killer cells and macrophages; stimulates other T cells to make IL-2 and interferon.

Lymphocyte: a class of white blood cells involved in acquired or specific immunity.

Macrophage: a class of white blood cells that migrates into the tissues. This phagocytic cell also acts as an antigen-presenting cell.

Major histocompatibility complex (MHC): a cluster of genes that encode cell surface molecules involved in T cell recognition of antigen. Class I MHC molecules are distributed on virtually all cells in the body. Class II MHC molecules are expressed on antigen-presenting cells and other activated cells. These molecules are associated with intense rejection of poorly matched organ grafts.

Memory: a characteristic of acquired immunity in which a second exposure to an antigen results in a faster, stronger, and longer-lasting response compared to the first encounter.

Memory cells: B and T cells that have been exposed to an antigen and are primed to give a memory response.

Mitogen: a substance that causes general proliferation (mitosis) of lymphocytes.

Monocyte: a white blood cell that becomes a macrophage when it leaves the blood.

Natural killer cell: a lymphocyte that is not a B or a T cell. It can kill virus infections and some cancer cells.

Neutrophil: the major class of granulocyte.

Phagocyte: a cell, such as a macrophage or neutrophil, that can engulf cells or other particles.

Respiratory burst: the increased oxidative metabolism that follows activation of phagocytic cells.

Suppressor T cell: a T lymphocyte that inhibits the function of other T cells.

T cell: a lymphocyte that may work as a helper T cell, a cytotoxic T cell, or a suppressor T cell. It characteristically has a molecular complex called CD3 on its surface, which is involved in stimulation after antigen recognition.

Thymocyte: an immature T cell in the thymus gland.

Thymus: a gland found near the heart in which T lymphocytes mature after being produced in the bone marrow.

Tolerance: a condition of induced specific immunologic nonresponsiveness.

Tumor necrosis factor: a cytokine, involved in inflammation, that can kill tumor cells.

Index

Cook, Richard, 82
Cooking
  of beans, 197–98
  of grains, 193–94
  of seaweed, 199–200
  of vegetables, 196
Copper
  benefits of, 54, 75
  deficiency of, 80
  effect on disease prevention, 224
  effect on immune system, 80
  nutritional sources of, 84
  synergy with zinc, 78–79
Cortinelin, 102
Cortisol
  effect of alcohol on, 290
  effect of depression on, 133, 150
  effect of exercise on, 120
  effect of relaxation on, 137
  effect of stress on, 36, 132, 274,
    281
  effect on immune system, 178
Coumarins, 113
Counselors (counseling), 140, 155,
  169
Cowania mexicana, 227
Crohn's disease, 123
Cruciferous vegetables, 113, 190
Cumin *(Cuminum cyminum),* 111,
  201, 206
Curcuma longa (turmeric), 110–11,
  201, 206, 226–27
Curcumin, 110, 226–27
Curry, 101
Cyclophosphamide, 109
Cysteine, 222
Cytokines, 14, 18–21, 22, 61, 129,
  241, 282, 299. *See also* Tumor
  necrosis factor
Cytotoxic T cells, 20, 24, 300

Davis, Maradee, 162–63
Deep breathing, 140–41, 190, 209
Dehydroepiandrosterone sulfate,
  137
Delta-tetrahydrocannabinol
  (DTHC), 175–76, 292

Depression
  effect of exercise on, 123
  effect of selenium on, 82
  effect of stress on, 133, 282
  effect on cortisol, 133, 150
  effect on disease prevention,
    150–51, 229–31
  treatment of, 208
Desserts, 202
Dexamethasone, 178
Diabetes, 28, 86, 129, 132
Diary writing, 135, 191. *See also*
  Journal writing
Diazepam, 294
Diet. *See also* Low-fat diet; Nutrition
  description of, 192–202
  menu suggestions for, 202–4,
    209–15
  nutrients in, 204–6
"Diet Balancer, The," 67
Dinner suggestions, 203–4
Dioxin, 179, 296
Disease, prevention of and recov-
  ery from, 3–4, 7. *See also*
  names of specific diseases
Distress, 134–35, 280
Dopamine, 142
Down syndrome, 254–55
Doxycycline, 178, 294
Dressings, dietary, 200–201
Drinking. *See* Alcohol
Dronabinol, 219
Drug abuse
  abstention from, 53, 191, 208
  effect on disease prevention,
    233, 291–93
  effect on fetus, 175
  effect on immune system, 171,
    174–76
  effect on zinc, 76, 256
DTHC (delta-tetrahydrocannabinol),
  175–76, 292
Dwarfism, 78

Ebola virus, 5
Echinacea *(Echinacea compositae),*
  106–7, 269